Beauty is more than skin deep... We all know our skin bears the brunt of environmental exposure, but what many don't realise is that the appearance of your skin is also an accurate reflection of your inner health. Unfortunately, we live in a society that conditions us to rely on pharmaceuticals and expensive cosmetics to disguise visible signs of ageing. In this book, Erica has provided you with sensible, easy-to-follow information that will help you to care for your health and appearance from the inside out. The good news is that it is never to late (or too early) to start taking care of your body. If you're looking tired and unwell, there's a very distinct chance that you are!

— Donna Aston, celebrity health and fitness trainer, author of *Fat or Fiction*, *Body Business*, *Stayin' Alive*, *Look Good Naked* and *Losing It*

Gorgeous Skin in 30 days compellingly shows how the typical Western diet promotes disease and accelerated ageing of the skin. In a scientifically accurate and easy-to-understand manner, Erica Angyal lays out the basic plan for good health and beautiful skin — a plan that mimics many features of the ancestral and native human diet.

— Loren Cordain, PhD, author of *The Paleo Diet*

With *Gorgeous Skin in 30 Days* Erica Angyal not only lays out the vital principals for healthy skin and a balanced lifestyle, but her safe detoxification plan and well researched nutritional program offer you natural and effective solutions for a healthier life in an increasingly toxic world.

— Dr Sandra Cabot MD, author of the *Liver Cleansing Diet*, *Boost Your Energy*, *Body Shaping Diet* and *The Healthy Liver and Bowel Book*

Our landmark study, published in 2001, which demonstrated that food and beverage intake could account for a significant part of skin wrinkling with age, has implications for general health as well. It is gratifying to know that promoters of public health, like Erica Angyal in *Gorgeous Skin in 30 Days* have ta........ .... cepts. In reality, however, food behaviours .... not without the pleasure of food.

— Professor Mark L. Wahlqvist AO, FTSE,

A blueprint for gorgeous skin, Erica Angyal provi....   ....g younger looking skin using the inside out approach. A must read for anyone who wants to keep the ageing process at bay.

— Tracy McWilliams, media personality and author of *Dress to Express* and *Revealing Your Inner Beauty*

Erica Angyal's program achieves results in such a way I've never seen from any beauty or diet book before. Many of the finalists at Miss Universe enter the competition with eating disorders, or they are too thin or overweight. After working with Erica on their diet and lifestyle for only a month, the transformation of their skin and bodies has been truly amazing. I highly recommend *Gorgeous Skin in 30 Days*. It is a must for every woman's beauty library.

— Inés Ligron, National Director Miss Universe, Japan

As a natural medicine practitioner specialising in clinical nutrition, I became aware of the importance of the appearance of the skin not only as a diagnostic tool, but as a yardstick to measure progress. The importance and essential connection between what we eat and how that reflects in the health and appearance of our skin has been largely ignored till now. Eloquently written and accurately researched, Erica Angyal's *Gorgeous Skin in 30 Days* captures the essence of that connection.

— Jayne Edmondson, natural medicine practitioner, Pro Health Clinic, Sydney

Our skin is the body's largest organ. It is literally everywhere ... and yet the amount of time we set aside to pay attention to this vital part of the magnificent machine that is the human body? Sometimes nil, sometimes a fleeting moment here and there. I am delighted to endorse Erica Angyal's book *Gorgeous Skin in 30 Days* — the information is invaluable.

— Dr John Tickell, author of *The Great Australian Diet*

Your skin is the window into the health and wellness of your body. You can't have great looking skin without a healthy body. Erica gives you the secrets of beauty from within. If you follow her dietary and lifestyle recommendations, your skin will show the difference within 30 days.

— Dr Barry Sears, author of *The Zone*

Erica Angyal makes it easy for anyone to understand how to have gorgeous skin — and she makes the point it is more lasting when done from the inside out. Changing the outside without the inside is no more enduring or functional than painting a 30-year-old car that doesn't have a motor; may look great, but will not move enough to satisfy. Those really interested in vital skin will find this book compelling and entertaining.

— Dr Mike Roizen, author of *RealAge* and *YOU: The Owner's Manual*

gorgeous skin

IN 30 DAYS

the natural anti-ageing plan
for radiant, youthful skin

erica angyal

Lothian
BOOKS

Important notice: The information and advice contained in this book is not intended to replace the services of a qualified health professional. Consult your doctor for health advice. Use of the information herein is beyond the control of the author and the publisher, who are not responsible for any problems arising from its application.

Thomas C. Lothian Pty Ltd
132 Albert Road, South Melbourne, Vic 3205
www.lothian.com.au

Copyright © Erica Angyal 2005
First published 2005

National Library of Australia
Cataloguing-in-Publication data:

Angyal, Erica.
Gorgeous skin in 30 days : the natural anti-ageing plan for radiant, youthful skin.

ISBN 0 7344 0833 1.

1. Skin — Care and hygiene. I. Title.

646.726

Editor: Sally Moss, Context Editorial
Cover design by Pip McConnel-Oats
Cover photograph by Kenji Maeji
Internal design and typesetting by David Constable
Colour reproduction by Print+Publish, Port Melbourne
Printed in Australia by Ligare

Preface

A gorgeous, healthy glow is top of the wish list for so many people, and we'll go to amazing lengths to achieve it. Yet we tend to focus on external strategies: cosmetics, skin-care products and even surgery. It's so hard not to be seduced by the beauty industry. We live in a society that glorifies youth, and we're besieged from all sides by beauty ads. We see them everyday on billboards, on the sides of buses, on magazine covers and in the mass media. With the world-wide cosmetic market worth four billion dollars annually and growing rapidly, it is no wonder we've become conditioned to think that beauty comes from outside and can be purchased in a cream or a lotion. Unfortunately, that's not the case.

Your skin is in a perpetual state of bloom, constantly repairing and replenishing itself through the creation of new cells, *from the inside*. But the condition of your skin depends on the quality of raw materials from which these cells are constructed. In other words, what you eat and drink produces the skin you reveal to the world. The way your skin looks is actually a direct portrayal of your diet and lifestyle. A gorgeous, glowing complexion reflects a state of great inner health, and the only way to get it is by working from within. There's no way around it!

The Gorgeous Skin program is a complete plan, based entirely on diet and lifestyle factors, for achieving radiant healthy skin and preventing premature ageing. This program represents the culmination of my lifelong passion for nutrition and my search to find ways to maintain health and beauty naturally.

My interest in the connection between the skin and nutrition goes back to the year I spent in Japan as an exchange student, when I lived in a small village on the southern island of Kyushu. After my arrival in Kyushu, I went through a complete change of diet and lifestyle almost overnight, and I discovered that what I ate had a huge impact on the appearance of my skin. Each day my Japanese hosts would prepare a breakfast of grilled fish, miso soup, seaweed and other delicacies and I noticed a remarkable improvement in the appearance of my skin. It was then that my interest in health and nutrition began, which eventually led me to study preventative medicine and become a nutritionist.

In my first few years as a nutritionist, I became increasingly aware of the connection between the appearance of my clients' skin and their diet. Often it didn't matter whether I was trying to improve a client's cholesterol levels or helping someone to shed a few unwanted kilograms, because a consistent result was a marked improvement in the colour and condition of their skin in response to changes in their diet. At the time I wasn't recommending a specific or tailored diet, but most of my clients followed similar advice: cutting back on processed foods, refined carbohydrates, sugar, caffeine, alcohol, fried foods and margarine, and increasing their intake of good fats from fish, olive oil and nuts, fresh fruit and vegetables, as well as increasing their sources of complex carbohydrates and protein. After several weeks following these dietary guidelines, I began to see subtle yet noticeable differences in their complexion. As the skin is our largest organ, and the only one visible to the eye, it's a valuable barometer for our internal health. Just by looking at my clients' skin, I could tell whether they had been following the diet I had prescribed.

Traditional Chinese Medicine (TCM) also gave me a good foundation to explore the link between the appearance of a person's skin and their general health. In TCM, the appearance of the face and tongue have been used as diagnostic tools for thousands of years. For instance, blackness under the eyes can indicate kidney problems; a yellowish hue to the skin can indicate spleen problems; a brown hue can indicate problems with the liver; and clear radiant skin is a mark of inner vitality.

As I began refining the diet I recommended to my clients, I was also reading and researching about the impact of food and supplements on skin and ageing. It was then that I discovered the startling results of research conducted Dr Mark Wahlqvist of Monash University in Melbourne. Dr Wahlqvist and his peers scientifically confirmed what I'd believed for years: not only does what we eat have an enormous impact on the appearance of our skin, it also affects how our skin ages.[1]

Each of the major factors involved in ageing, such as excess free radical production, inflammation, declining hormone levels and damage to DNA, can be positively affected by what we eat and how we live. By providing the correct nutrition that the cells in the body need to operate at the optimum level for health and vitality through the Gorgeous Skin program, we can help to slow down the ageing process in our skin as well as our body.

We all want to look good no matter what our age, and when we look good, we really do feel our best. As there is an intrinsic relationship between inner health and outer beauty, the goal of looking good doesn't have to be about vanity or an obsession with youth. Our skin is a window to our internal health and it provides a clue to the speed at which we are ageing internally.

Even if you are already blessed with beautiful skin, you will still benefit from the Gorgeous Skin program and you'll feel fantastic. A great diet with a balanced healthy lifestyle, along with external skin care and protection, *can* and *will* help to slow the ageing process of your skin, proving that health and beauty really do go hand in hand.

Erica Angyal
Tokyo, Japan

Acknowledgements

Although writing is an individual sport, creating a book is a real team effort. I am deeply grateful to everyone who has made this book possible, including:

My US agent, Jeff Herman, who believed in the book from the beginning. My Australian agent Tara Wynne from Curtis Brown, who has been nothing short of fantastic. My managing editor at Lothian Books Magnolia Flora for her great enthusiasm, vision and commitment and to Sally Moss for her wonderful editing. My dear friends Pip McConnel-Oats for her beautiful design work on the cover and colour pages and Kenji Maeji for the superb cover shot and recipe photos and Bibi for her yoga illustrations. Many thanks also to the outstanding Lothian Books team, including Georgina Way and Peter Lothian, and the entire sales and marketing, and production staffs. I feel so blessed to have such talented people around me.

I'm especially indebted to Mike Merrill, for reviewing and editing countless drafts and being such amazing support. Special thanks to Jayne Edmondson for her contribution of recipes, and for all her invaluable assistance and advice. I also wish to thank Xavier Destribats of the Grand Hyatt Tokyo for his kind assistance and Executive Chefs Josef Budde and Yasuhiro Toshida for preparing many of the fabulous recipe shots. Thanks also to Tony Scimonello, chef/caterer in Tokyo, for his help fine-tuning all the recipes.

A big thanks to everyone else who has contributed in so many ways, including Jessica Hollander, treasured friend, for her amazing eye and editing skills; Barbara Chappell, Libby Allen, Ray Gordon, Linda Sherman, Inés Ligron, Monica Levy, Bibi, Tracy McWilliams, and countless others who have inspired and assisted in so many ways.

Many thanks to the pioneering authors, researchers, nutritionists, doctors and patients everywhere whose work has helped shape my overall perspective and contributed to this book, including Dr Barry Sears, Dr Loren Cordain, Dr Michael Roizen, Dr Vincent Giampapa, Dr Jeffrey Bland, Dr Andrew Weil, Jack Challem, Dr Jennie Brand-Miller, Professor Mark Wahlqvist, Donna Aston, Leslie Kenton, Udo Erasmus, Mike Curley, Dr Tony Goh, Dr Sandra Cabot, Edward Obaidey, Ross Penman, Sylvia Deitch and Jayne Edmondson.

I am truly fortunate to have such a wonderful family. To my mum and dad, Suzie and Peter, my brother Brendan, I am so grateful for all your love, inspiration, wisdom and support.

And finally to my hero and love of my life, Wolfgang, who made it all possible: thank you for your unwavering support, love and encouragement.

Contents

Introduction

Why We Should Love Our Skin

'Flawless skin is the most universally desired human feature.'
— Desmond Morris, renowned scientist and author

Gorgeous, glowing skin really is the ultimate fashion accessory; it never goes out of style and we all desire it, no matter what our age. According to a recent poll in the US magazine *Allure* an astounding 88 per cent of women rate having beautiful skin as more desirable than having a great body![2] And research conducted at the University College London found that men, when judging attractiveness in women, also focus on a woman's face more than on her figure.[3] Ratings for sexiness and healthiness were highest for the images that showed attractive faces and luminous skin, even on women who were not 'thin' by any measure. The desire for physical beauty is deeply ingrained in the human psyche; it doesn't matter whether we're old or young, male or female. More and more Australian men are buying into the beauty experience too, with men's skin care and cosmetic ranges experiencing double-digit growth. Cosmetic brands such as Ella Baché say that men comprise as much as 40 per cent of their salon customers.[4]

The quest for beauty isn't only a Western obsession; it's a global phenomenon and a primal one, too. In fact, our obsession with beautiful skin goes all the way back to the way our brains are wired — and it's all about appearing youthful and vital. The flush of the cheeks and a subtle glow send out a subconscious signal of youth, fertility and vitality and they're a marker of attraction for a potential partner. This is a major reason why women of all ages (and, increasingly, men) go all-out to maintain beautiful skin for life, and in doing so join in the universal obsession with a flawless complexion.

The fact is we do create impressions because of how we look. But these days our society worships beauty and is obsessed with youth like no other time in history. Worldwide, each year women shell out a staggering 246 billion dollars on youth, beauty and sex appeal in the form of cosmetics and skincare products (and who knows what the figures are for men!).

The beauty business is enormous; worldwide, it churns out thirty thousand advertisements a day and besieges us from all sides. We're bombarded with gorgeous, glossy images of perfection in advertising and the media. Shots of models gracing the covers of fashion magazines are virtually all airbrushed or digitally enhanced, making it impossible to achieve the mythical levels of beauty we see around us. And don't think you can escape its influence!

Luminous, lineless skin forever? You only have to witness the boom in the anti-ageing industry to see that we've become more and more obsessed with cheating old age. Few of us would resist selling our souls for the promise of everlasting youth. Actresses advancing in their years seem perpetually youthful and gorgeous, and in the process have redefined ageing.

But you would have thought that if anti-ageing skincare was so effective, surgery and other medical interventions wouldn't be necessary, at least not in the second and third decades of life. Yet, in the United States anyway, cosmetic surgery is enjoying a phenomenal surge in demand. According to the American Society of Plastic and Reconstructive Surgeons, about 8.3 million cosmetic surgery procedures were performed in the United States in 2003 — an increase of almost 36 per cent since 2001. Of these women, an astounding forty per cent were under the age of thirty. Even more astonishing is that the overall number of cosmetic procedures has increased 228 per cent since 1997. Cosmetic surgery can be very deceptive, though. Because if you decide to go down the surgery route, even for so-called subtle procedures you'll no doubt look younger on the outside, but your body will still be steadily ageing on the inside. So it's a major trap — youthful-looking skin on the outside but a steadily ageing body on the inside. Plus, you won't *feel* younger, either!

Simply put, ageing isn't just the unfolding of a genetic timetable. Ageing of your skin has a lot to do with the damage you do on the inside through poor food and lifestyle choices. Your skin, like everything else about you, is a product of the marriage between your genes and your environment. You don't have control over your genes, so no amount of skincare can guarantee you the perfect skin. But you do have a lot of control over your environment! In fact, accelerated ageing is due more to our diets and lifestyles than to our genes. A great diet and a healthy, balanced lifestyle can and will help to slow the ageing process. And given the right ingredients (nutrients from both food and supplements) your skin has a remarkable ability to rejuvenate. So time, in fact, is not your greatest enemy!

Your skin truly is a window into your internal world, and it provides a clue to the speed at which you are ageing internally: ageing skin is a signpost of an ageing body. Once you understand why your diet has such a profound impact on your skin and how you age, you'll be motivated, for the sake of vanity (if not longevity and overall wellness), to make some major changes to your diet and lifestyle. A really good diet along with a balanced, healthy lifestyle — combined, of course, with exterior care and protection — can and will help slow down the ageing process in your skin. Whatever you do for the health of your skin will improve the health of your body, and whatever you do for the health of your body will improve the health and appearance of your skin. The best news is that the healthy glow of gorgeous skin reflects a healthy body.

Genetics aside, it does take work to maintain great skin at every age. There are no shortcuts to naturally gorgeous skin — vitality and good health really do radiate from the inside out. The best line of defence is a nutrient-rich diet. This should be combined with anti-ageing supplements; some form of regular relaxation (such as meditation or yoga) plus moderate exercise; and avoiding the major 'skin sins' (such as too much sun, sugar and cigarette smoke).

Beginning right now, you have complete control over making healthy lifestyle choices that ultimately control how well and how fast you age. If you take care of yourself, you'll regain the radiance and vitality of your skin and keep it for life.

1

Three Steps to Gorgeous Skin

How the Program Works

The Gorgeous Skin program is a plan not only for your skin but also for your body and mind — it will help you look fabulous and feel fantastic. Its benefits are twofold: achieving truly great skin and preventing premature ageing. By nourishing, repairing, and protecting your skin, you will also be restoring health to your body. Think about it. The cells of your vital organs, like those of your skin, need a constant supply of oxygen, water and nutrients too!

The Gorgeous Skin program is a three-tiered plan, structured as follows:

Step 1 — Diet
Step 2 — Boosters (supplements and detoxification)
Step 3 — Lifestyle (exercise and relaxation).

Step 1 – Eat yourself gorgeous

We've all heard the cliché 'You are what you eat.' The truth is, what you eat does affect how you look — not only today but also especially down the road. Because absolutely everything you eat (and don't eat, for that matter) will affect the quality of your skin. That's why the first goal of the Gorgeous Skin program is to provide your skin with optimum nutrition through diet.

The health and beauty of every part of your skin — the epidermis (outer layer), dermis (inner layer) and subcutaneous layer (fatty layer) — depend on the quality of nutrients received from your bloodstream. And the journey these nutrients make is a long one! For your skin cells to look their absolute best they need a nutrient-rich, highly oxygenated blood supply, plus plenty of mineral building blocks and essential fats.

In an international study of eating patterns and skin ageing, researchers found that both fair-skinned and dark-skinned people who ate plenty of healthy foods (such as green leafy vegetables, beans, olive oil, nuts and fish) were less prone to wrinkling than those who ate lots of butter, margarine, red meat, fatty processed meats, sugar, soft drinks, cordials and refined carbohydrates.[5] So your most powerful beauty tools for achieving lifelong health and beauty are in fact the knife, the fork and the spoon!

Step 2 — Add some beauty boosters

The second tier of the Gorgeous Skin program starts with the inclusion of supplements. These are an important part of the overall picture, as they really help maximise the effects of skin rejuvenation. Because your skin is such an efficient barrier, and its outer layer has no blood supply, we need to supply all the necessary nutrients and other vital materials to the deeper layers, where the cells are nourished.

Supplements definitely can't replace a great diet, nor can they compensate for a poor diet. Food is a far superior form of nutrition and whole foods contribute to your health in myriad other ways. Nutritional supplements do, however, give your diet a great boost, and they can be a powerful extra weapon in the fight against premature ageing.

Each of the supplements recommended in this book will provide your body with everything needed to help stimulate new cell growth, repair vital skin structures, reduce oxidative stress and increase circulation. Together these effects will give you a radiance and a dewy, supple skin that you haven't seen in years.

The Gorgeous Skin plan also includes a three-day detoxification program. Ideally, if we lived in a pollution-free environment, ate only pure, organically grown, unprocessed foods, drank clean fresh water, exercised regularly and avoided all stress, pollutants and chemicals, our skin would be luminous and we would have vital health! And we certainly wouldn't need to detox. But the big problem these days is that toxins and metabolic wastes work their way into our bodies faster than they can be eliminated. A radiant, clear complexion begins with proper nutrition; efficient digestion and assimilation of nutrients by the body; and, last but not least, regular elimination. So for the ultimate goal of gorgeous skin, we should ideally improve our digestion and elimination while adding the healthiest nutrition.

A short detox is like an internal spring clean for your body at the deep cellular level. It gives your digestive system, including your liver, a well-deserved rest, so your body can focus on clearing out toxins such as environmental chemicals, which you have accumulated in your cells and tissues over the years, and internal toxins (preservatives, pesticides, caffeine, alcohol, additives, and so on). The three-day detoxification program is designed to trigger a gentle yet effective detoxification and to kick-start your 30-day Gorgeous Skin program.

Step 3 — Get some lifestyle protection

The third tier of the program is to modify your lifestyle to include what I've called 'protectors': they're an important part of your complete natural anti-ageing strategy. Because, even if you follow the Gorgeous Skin diet to a T, unless you incorporate these 'protectors' into your life you could still fail to slow the ageing process. They include deep restful sleep, moderate exercise, deep breathing, and a relaxation method such as yoga or meditation. Each of these has a profound impact on your hormones through your endocrine system and on reducing the activity of highly reactive and potentially destructive molecules known as free radicals, thereby greatly improving how your skin looks and ages.

Relaxation such as meditation and yoga really can help you stay youthful and vital. Countless studies show that people who do some form of deep relaxation such as yoga or meditation look younger and are biologically younger than those who don't! This is because deep relaxation can help switch on your body's calming nervous system, which ultimately leads to a shift from the production of age-promoting stress hormones, such as cortisol, to calming, age-protecting ones. When we're healthy internally — physically, mentally and emotionally — our outer beauty, including our skin, really glows.

The bigger picture

The 30-day Gorgeous Skin program puts all the principles for achieving lifelong health and beauty into a complete one-month diet and lifestyle program. It's a revolutionary nutritional program that includes all the skin 'super foods' to help reduce inflammation, rejuvenate your skin and revitalise your health. It's an appealing, easy-to-follow plan, so you won't have to count kilojoules, portion sizes or carbohydrate grams, or keep track of each snack along the way. Towards the end of the book, you'll find many of the recipes for the menus in the 30-day Gorgeous Skin program. But you're welcome to include others that you know or to search through cookbooks or on the Internet for additional recipes and food ideas — you can indulge your creativity, but just remember to stick to the beauty foods listed at the end of Chapter 8. Each meal in the program contains a balance of quality protein and non-starchy low-GI (glycaemic index) carbohydrates, along with generous amounts of good fats. This ensures stable blood sugar and insulin levels, as well as balanced hormone levels — keys to youthful, radiant skin.

In addition, you'll find (in Chapter 9) a 28-day plan for special occasions, including that all-important wedding. Eating well and healthily in the weeks leading up to your special day will give you a radiant glow that no skincare or makeup can! The Gorgeous Skin plan for special occasions is designed to be super easy to follow, as the last thing you need is extra stress preparing for such an event.

But the book also tells you what not to eat and what not to do if you want to achieve gorgeous skin. The logic is simple: there's no point in putting one foot on the brake against ageing if you have the other foot firmly planted on the accelerator! Excessive sun and cigarettes aren't the only culprits when it comes to premature ageing! Chapter 6 will show you how many of the foods that we eat on a daily basis not only have an impact on the general appearance of our skin but also on how fast we age. You may be shocked at how many of your food choices are responsible for accelerated ageing. In fact, many of the foods we unthinkingly put in our mouths everyday create a combat zone for our skin.

Along with the 'skin sins', I'll explain why avoiding the 'youthful risk takers' — such as stress, smoking, yo-yo dieting, excesses of alcohol, caffeine and sun exposure — can add years to your looks and your life. We all know that the sun, especially the harsh Australian sun, ages our skin rapidly, powerfully and cumulatively. But you may be surprised to hear that stress can have devastating long-term consequences for your skin! Stress triggers the production of a number of stress hormones including one called cortisol. In small amounts it's harmless, but pump out too much cortisol and your blood sugar levels soar, which in turn increases insulin levels — a major age accelerator. High levels of cortisol can also thin the skin, promote inflammation and cause a whole host of other skin problems! Preserving youthful levels of key hormones and reducing cortisol levels is key to keeping a gorgeous, youthful complexion forever.

It's important to note that the Gorgeous Skin program will complement any other skincare program, skin surgery or skin rejuvenation procedure that you may embark upon. Even if you have chosen cosmetic surgery, you won't maintain a youthful appearance unless you back it up with looking after yourself through a great diet and control of molecular damage, inflammation and other accelerators. In fact, a forward-thinking plastic surgeon from the United States, Dr James Carraway, has been quoted as saying 'nutrition is the single most important factor for my patients'. Dr Carraway has a full-time nutritionist on staff and counsels his patients in nutrition, supplements, stress management and exercise.[6] Remember that surgery can do nothing to slow, stop or reverse the ageing process inside our bodies.

Your skin, with the right diet and care, has an amazing ability to rejuvenate at any age. It's never too late to get started. By following the food, supplement and lifestyle strategies outlined in this book, along with avoiding the 'skin sins', it will make a huge difference to your skin and to your life! Be persistent: You may notice subtle changes in your skin within a few days, but lasting results can sometimes take up to three or four weeks. And the improvement will continue as long as you follow the program. Don't forget a radiant complexion is a prime indicator of your overall health. Within 30 days you'll look younger and feel healthier than you have in years.

The Gorgeous Skin program will show you that healthy living can be the best cosmetic of all. Your face will look rested, rejuvenated and revitalised. Your skin's natural glow will return as capillary circulation and lymphatic drainage improve. Skin blemishes, blotches and spots will diminish or disappear. The whites of your eyes will become whiter; dark circles will diminish. Your skin texture will appear smoother and softer, and fine lines will appear less noticeable. Consider the 30 days of the program as a gift to your health, beauty and wellbeing for now, and for life.

Lastly, why a 30-day program? This is the average time it takes new skin cells to push to the surface of the epidermis. So when you look at your skin, you're actually looking at the result of your last thirty-day skin renewal cycle. If you don't like what you see, you know you haven't been taking proper care of yourself. With great nutrition and a healthy, balanced lifestyle your skin will rebuild itself and it's your best bet for achieving lifelong health and beauty.

2

The Basics

Building Beauty from Within

From the outside, your skin may look like a 'passive' organ that's sitting idle until it gets cleansed, moisturised or cared for from the outside. But beautiful skin is so much more than skin deep. The outer layer of skin that's visible to the eye is actually only a small part of what's really happening with our skin. The real action is taking place directly below and from deeper within. Underneath, your body is working hard at performing hundreds of tasks simultaneously to keep your skin healthy. Apart from fending off a daily beating from environmental assaults like UV rays, pollution and chemical toxins, your skin is processing over 300 million skin cells at any one time, working around the clock to shield you from invading micro-organisms, regulating body temperature and providing you with a glove-like waterproof covering for your body. And on top of all that, your skin is also busy shielding you from the inner assault that comes mainly from what you eat and from your lifestyle!

For as long as people (mainly women but increasingly men) have been looking after their looks, they've focused almost exclusively on external strategies. We put on creams, serums, moisturisers and make-up; we exfoliate our skin and protect it from the sun's scorching rays. We have facials and indulge in other feel-good beauty treatments that promise beautiful skin. Many of these have great effects, at least temporarily, but we generally don't look beyond these external strategies. Yet, with a few genetically blessed exceptions, for most of us, those rosy, glowing cheeks don't just happen!

Sure, technology is becoming more and more sophisticated and the anti-ageing claims are becoming more seductive, with an ever-increasing array of anti-ageing products that promise to 'erase the first signs of ageing', 'help minimise visible lines and wrinkles' and 'see visible results after just eight days'! One of the most amazing aspects of the cosmetics and skincare industry is that the Australian regulatory body the Therapeutic Goods Administration (TGA) does not require companies to prove their claims. This means that skin-care companies get to say just about anything they want about their products without any substantiation or proof whatsoever.

What skincare products can do is nurture the *surface* of your skin, plump up the *outer layer*, and make your skin *look* more hydrated and moist, but the vast majority can't penetrate deeper. Any good basic moisturiser will temporarily make skin look and feel more supple and youthful, but most won't do anything to prevent ageing or have an effect on the deeper layers of your skin where wrinkles are formed.

Your skin is designed as a barrier not a sponge, and despite all those diagrams you see showing creams penetrating deep into the skin, it's very difficult to go beyond the thin outer layer. When you understand your skin you'll realise that the vast majority of products can do little more than cleanse, protect and polish. So let's take a quick look at your skin.

The skin you're in

Your skin has three distinct layers: the epidermis, the dermis, and the subcutaneous or fat layer (also sometimes called the hypodermis).

When we look in the mirror what we see is our epidermis, a thin outer layer. It's the first barrier between you and the environment

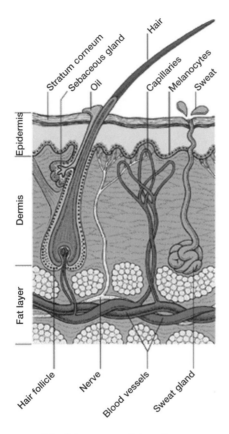

and it acts like a suit of amour, protecting you from environmental assaults including UV radiation, free radicals, heat and cold, pollution, water loss, toxic chemicals and infectious organisms. This is the layer that also regenerates — new cells are continuously made as the outer layer dies and wears away. The condition of your epidermis actually determines how 'fresh' your skin looks and how well it absorbs and holds moisture.

Your epidermis, in turn, is composed of four thin layers. The very bottom layer is where your cells are continually dividing to produce millions of plump new skin cells daily. These cells are made from fatty acids, amino acids and other vital substances provided by your bloodstream, so they start off looking like plump round grapes. But by the time they work their way up to the very outer layer, they've flattened out, died and start to resemble dried-out raisins! It's here at the *stratum corneum*, the very outer layer of your epidermis, that these dead skin cells are continually shedding. Your epidermal layer doesn't have a blood supply, though, which means there is no supply of nutrients to feed and nourish your newly formed skin cells. In a unique piece of engineering, the basal layer sits just above your skin's next layer down, the dermis, and benefits from a nourishment and oxygen exchange with this layer.

Most skincare products work on the *stratum corneum*, even though it's composed of dead cells. When you plump up this surface layer it distributes light more evenly, creating the appearance of smoother, more radiant skin. But in order to actually improve the condition of your skin and have an impact on your collagen and elastin, the active ingredients of a product would need to penetrate your epidermis and find their way into your dermis, which isn't the easiest of tasks. According to Dr Richard Glogau, clinical professor of dermatology at the University of California, San Francisco, it's very difficult for a product's active ingredients to penetrate the junction between the top layers of skin and the dermis. 'The whole point of the epidermis is to prevent things on the outside (including collagen) from getting in,' Glogau says. 'I see a lot of creams that demonstrate activity in a test tube, but it's a big leap of logic to say that they'll have the same effect topically on the skin, because the ingredients may never get past the epidermis.'[7]

The next layer down is your dermis, and this is the layer that generally works the hardest to keep your skin healthy. Your dermis is responsible for your skin's structural integrity, elasticity and resilience and it also acts like a supportive mattress for your epidermis. It's a very dynamic layer which is also in constant turnover.

This is also the layer where all the action happens: it's where wrinkles arise and develop; and where you find collagen, elastin and moisture-holding molecules such as hyaluronic acid — the three main factors that keep your skin firm, moist and youthful. In other words, it determines the tone of your skin. The skin cells in the dermis actually regenerate new collagen while the old collagen is being broken down, a process that happens continually but slows with age as well as imposed factors such as smoking, exposure to sun, stress, and poor nutrition.

Your dermis is where your cells do the work to keep your skin fit. And unlike your epidermis, it is composed entirely of living cells.

Your dermis is also rich in capillaries — tiny blood vessels that bring fresh nutrients and oxygen vital for new cell production. These nutrients push their way from the dermis into your epidermis where they keep your skin cells healthy. The capillaries also remove carbon dioxide and other metabolic wastes from your skin cells. As well, this dermal layer contains blood and lymph vessels, sebaceous and sweat glands, hair follicles and touch and pain receptors.

The last and innermost layer of your skin is the subcutaneous layer. It acts as a 'shock absorber' for your skin and functions like a pillow, cushioning your internal organs, holding in body heat and giving contour to your skin. This layer also contains a network of blood vessels, lymph vessels and nerves. Fat cells, collagen, and elastin reside here too. As you age, the subcutaneous layer thins, giving you a more angular appearance.

Resist the cosmeceutical con

The condition of the surface of your skin (the epidermis) reflects what's happening underneath. Remember, this layer that you cleanse and moisturise — the epidermal layer — doesn't have a direct blood supply. Most dermatologists agree that moisturisers temporarily give dry skin the appearance of softness and moisture, plumping out wrinkles by adding water. But once the moisturiser is absorbed, the effect goes away.

Unfortunately moisturisers don't become more effective the more they cost. According to Dr Tom Rohrer, dermatologist at the Boston University School of Medicine in the United States, 'this is because, despite their baffling array of ingredients, they work basically the same way: They trap water that's already inside the skin, as opposed to adding moisture from the outside. Moisturisers help seal things off and allow less moisture to escape.'[8]

Sadly, the news on wrinkle reducers and anti-ageing creams isn't any better. The biggest misconception about anti-ageing creams is the term 'anti-ageing'. Moisturisers that claim to get rid of wrinkles or reduce the appearance of age really don't — all they do is plump up the skin momentarily, despite manufacturers' claims of clinical trials to the contrary. It's this temporary plumping you can see in the 'before' and 'after' photos. But any other basic moisturiser does this just as well. The bottom line is that most moisturisers don't penetrate your skin.[9]

And the picture isn't much rosier for antioxidant creams and the newer cosmeceutical topicals. These are non-prescription creams, gels and lotions that promise dramatic results. They often include a variety of antioxidants and anti-inflammatory botanicals. But they are not controlled by the TGA (nor the FDA in America), which means that manufacturers aren't required to conduct clinical trials to demonstrate a product's efficacy or safety. In Japan, by contrast, these active ingredients are called 'quasi-drugs' and must be proven mild and safe. In general, the makers of cosmeceuticals can't make claims that their products reverse or prevent the effects of ageing but their marketing can include statements about benefits to skin appearance or texture.

A number of studies have found that antioxidants do have a protective effect when applied topically before the skin's exposure to UV rays. But the jury is out as to whether they do actually prevent the ageing of skin. According to Dr Jeffrey Blumberg, Chief of Antioxidants Research at Tufts University in the United States, 'despite the proliferation of skin-care products that contain antioxidants there is no conclusive scientific evidence that antioxidants really prevent wrinkles, nor is there any information about how much antioxidant(s) or exactly which one(s) has to be present in a product to have an effect'.[10] According to Albert M. Kligman, MD, PhD, who coined the term *cosmeceuticals* and, more than twenty years ago, discovered the benefits of topical tretinoin (Retin-A), 'Ninety per cent of those products have no effects whatsoever.'[11] The fact is that most of the age-fighting products available lack scientific data to support their claims.

Despite this lack of hard evidence, fashion magazines and cosmetics companies have heralded the elimination of free-radical damage as the fountain of youth and cosmeceuticals and antioxidant creams as the answer. And we all get so swept up in the hype. Who can resist a product that promises a radiant glow and a turning back of the clock! Yet there are only a few products backed by clear-cut medical evidence that show they reduce wrinkles. Retin-A and its close relatives are among them. Sunscreen is also referred to as an anti-ageing agent as it provides protection from ageing UV rays. The rest are clever studies, which are mostly funded by the very companies that produce the products.

According to Anita Roddick, founder of the worldwide Body Shop chain of stores, ninety-nine per cent of the cost of cosmetics goes into the packaging, marketing and advertising! So it's all pretty much hype and clever marketing. Dr Danné Montagu-King, an American doctor with a line of face peels and anti-cellulite treatments says, 'ninety-five per cent of the beauty industry is fake and anyone can challenge me on it'.[12] And if this isn't enough to convince you, think about this. There are at least ten thousand different anti-ageing products currently on the market. You have to wonder why, if any one of them was the answer, they don't just sell that!

So there really aren't any miracle moisturisers, magic lotions or rejuvenating creams. And none of them can turn back the clock. Anti-ageing begins on a cellular level, not on the surface of your skin as many skincare companies would love you to believe. Short of surgery, there isn't a magical elixir for eternal youth! So next time you get seduced by an amazing claim of a product reducing the visible signs of ageing, ask the salesperson how the product works at a cellular level. If they can't explain it in logical terms that you understand, walk out the door. Or better yet, ask for published independent research on that product. And if they can't produce this, still walk out the door.

Vitamin C is another false saviour worth mentioning here. Despite its shaky medical standing, plenty of women worship at the shrine of C. Theoretically, vitamin C, an antioxidant, prevents and reverses ageing by mopping up free radicals responsible for skin damage. However, it's not clear whether vitamin C can penetrate the skin, no matter what its formulation and advertising claims. Even if vitamin C molecules do get through the skin, there's insufficient evidence that they do much, dermatologists say.[13] Another major problem is delivery of these ingredients. The ingredients have to remain stable in the bottle and then must penetrate the skin under a variety of conditions. Which isn't the easiest of tasks.

The male skin advantage

When it comes to skin, men have an advantage over women and it's all to do with testosterone, the predominately male hormone that gives men an enviably thicker epidermis. In fact the total skin thickness in men is about 25 per cent greater than in women! Testosterone also makes men's skin tougher and less sensitive. In general, male skin is oilier, with larger pores and a richer blood supply, plus they have more collagen and elastin.

As we grow older, the differences become even more dramatic. Later in middle age, men's testosterone levels and women's oestrogen levels drop, resulting in thinner, more fragile skin for both sexes. In women, however, the drop in hormone activity is more dramatic and has a greater effect, causing skin to become thinner and drier.

However, despite the better 'handicap', most men usually lose out on the relative advantages due to their more careless general attitude towards diet and lifestyle. Men's skin is also subject to the same daily stresses, the effects of pollution and the harsh Australian sun, so it needs just the same level of attention, care and protection. For that reason any man following the Gorgeous Skin diet and lifestyle program can benefit just as much. So men take note: men and women find their partners more attractive if they have great skin.

Nutrients: your most powerful beauty tools

So if beautiful skin doesn't come in a bottle, where do the secrets of flawless skin and ageless beauty lie? First your skin needs to be healthy in order to be beautiful. Health and beauty are intrinsically linked. When was the last time you saw a truly unhealthy person with a perfect complexion and a healthy glow? Your skin's lustre, tone and vibrancy are intimately related to what you eat, as your skin cells are in constant turnover and your whole outer layer is regenerating each month. No amount of makeup can conceal the telltale signs of a sallow, blemished or lacklustre complexion. Your skin cells need a highly oxygenated, nutrient-rich blood supply and plenty of mineral building blocks, great protein and essential fats to look their absolute best. Of course a good moisturiser and a sunscreen (non-chemical where possible) are still a must, but remember that your skin is actually designed as a barrier, so the way your surface skin looks is really determined much deeper, in the dermis — at the deep cellular level. The solution is to support and nourish your skin from deep down, where it begins.

What your skin gets or doesn't get from within is primarily determined by what you do or do not put into your body! Cell turnover and collagen production are ongoing processes that need to be maintained at an optimal level for your skin to look its absolute best. This can only be achieved by continuously feeding your skin cells internally with food and nutrients that repair, restore and protect it. So a subtle glow and a rosy sheen shout of a health and vibrancy that can only come from within.

There's no way around it — great nutrition and a healthy, balanced lifestyle are absolutely critical to building healthy skin cells. The foods you choose can be the difference between a gorgeous, youthful, luminous complexion and a dull, blemished or prematurely aged skin. This chapter shows how you can build beautiful skin from the inside out and how to minimise the effects of ageing by what you eat on a daily basis.

In introducing your beauty tools, let me start by alerting you to the number one enemy from within: the typical Western diet! It's high in sugar, refined carbohydrates, caffeine, alcohol, processed foods and bad fats, yet deficient in so many key nutrients. It's also chock full of high fat, preserved, pesticide-laden and chemically treated food plus free-radical formers such as margarine, sugar, white flour and alcohol. It emphasises frying, barbecuing and other cooking methods that exponentially drive up the free-radical count. Most significantly, it's dangerously deficient in antioxidant-rich free-radical fighting fruits and vegetables. So how does your skin stand a fighting chance of looking its absolute best if you don't feed it all the nutrients that it needs for repair and rejuvenation? It doesn't.

It's a sure bet that you're going to be deficient in a whole stack of nutrients. You might have acne from the hydrogenated oils in chocolate bars and chips and your skin may look puffy, sallow and unpolished from a lack of essential fats and too many processed and refined foods. Even if you tend to fall somewhere in the middle — trying your best to eat vegetables and salads, while indulging in the occasional pizza and junk food — you probably think your skin could look better.

I know it's often really difficult to make healthy choices. It's so much easier to munch on potato chips, biscuits, chocolate or take-away than to prepare a healthy snack that's loaded with skin-protecting antioxidants, vitamins, minerals, healthy fats and phytonutrients. A burger versus a fresh salad with salmon? A cake filled with refined flour, sugar and margarine for dessert, or fresh fruit? A tasty snack that lasts for a few moments or … vitality, health and beautiful clear skin. Make no mistake, eating your way to beauty does take a little more time and effort, but when you make the healthy choices, the rewards for both your skin and your health are enormous. And even small changes to your diet can make a huge difference to your complexion. The freshest fruit and vegetables, lean protein from cold-water fish and free-range poultry, complex carbohydrates (non-starchy and low GI) and good fats from nuts and cold-pressed olive oil are the best 'cosmetics'. The great news is that the food outlined in this chapter can also help prevent cross-linking of collagen, which is responsible for wrinkle and line formation, and it can even help repair the damage to your skin cells that comes with ageing.

So what kinds of foods are sensational for our skin? Let's look at the five groups that matter.

The power of fruits and vegetables

Fruits and vegetables are *numero uno* for your skin. Of all foods, fruits and vegetables are the most nutrient dense, meaning they contain the most vitamins and minerals per kilojoule rating.

Specifically, they are natural sources of vitamin C and E, which are health-promoting antioxidants, and are natural powerhouses of bioflavonoids. Vitamin C and bioflavonoids found in natural foods (such as the whitish inner membranes in grapefruit) ensure the health of the tiny capillaries that supply nutrients to your skin's cells, and in doing so they protect your skin from fragile or broken veins, bruising and early wrinkling.

Your capillaries are vital pipelines for your skin cells. When they are weak or are not working efficiently, your skin's cells don't receive all the oxygen and nutrients they need. This can also lead to inefficient elimination of wastes; stagnation in your tissues; and sallow, puffy, prematurely aged or dull skin. In addition vitamin C and bioflavonoids help keep skin young by protecting collagen fibres. Your skin requires the constant synthesis of new collagen to remain firm and youthful — without adequate vitamin C, your collagen fibres in the deepest layers (the dermis) can suffer damage.

Fruits and vegetables are also loaded with the 'beauty minerals' — silica, magnesium, calcium and sulphur, and with the minerals zinc and selenium. Sulphur is particularly important for beautiful skin. It must be present in every cell, as it's responsible for pulling in nutrition and removing waste from your cells. This is what is called osmosis. For great skin you need to have good osmosis.

What's more, fruits and vegetables pack a powerful punch of protective plant nutrients called phytonutrients or phytochemicals (phytos). Phytonutrients are particularly important for keeping your skin youthful and gorgeous as they act as antioxidants, fending off free-radical damage. Certain phytonutrients can also help protect your skin from sun damage and UV radiation, which they achieve by boosting your skin's natural defences. Finally, fruits and vegetables also create an optimal alkaline pH state in the body and, as an added bonus, they help keep your body toxin-free via their all-important role in detoxification.

Fearless phytos

Of all of the fantastic properties of fruits and vegetables, it's the phytonutrients that we're most interested in here. These powerful antioxidants, found only in plants — fruits, vegetables, nuts, grains and legumes — are our strongest weapon against ageing free radicals. By 'scavenging' these free radicals, the phytos prevent oxidative damage to our cells. These active plant molecules are what give plants their colour, flavour and natural disease resistance. For example, tomatoes have lycopene, garlic has allicin and blueberries have proanthocyanidins. All of these contribute to our health and beauty in so many ways. Research shows that phytonutrients, working together with other nutrients found in fruits, vegetables and nuts, reduce the risk of just about every single lifestyle-induced disease and can help slow the ageing process. Antioxidant phytonutrients number in the thousands and, though they act as powerful anti-oxidants, there are myriad ways in which they further reduce oxidation caused by free radicals. According to Dr Timothy Smith, author of *Renewal: the Anti-aging Revolution*, 'One of your most powerful anti-aging strategies is to make phytonutrient-rich food the centerpiece of your diet.'[14]

Your skin is at the front line of exposure to free radicals. Not only do your skin cells have to contend directly with environmental toxins such as pollution, cigarette smoke and UV radiation but they also suffer from the same oxidative stress as other cells in your body. It's estimated that each and every cell in your body gets at least ten thousand oxidative hits per day! Amazingly, your cells can withstand this type of punishment as long as your antioxidant guard is up. But when your antioxidant intake falls below par, free radicals gain the upper hand. A few thousand hits here, a few thousand hits there, and pretty soon you're dealing with major cell damage.

The key thing to remember is that excessive free radicals are synonymous with damage. They damage everything they come in contact with, insidiously and silently. But what does this mean for your skin? Free radicals can damage three major sites in your skin:

What are free radicals?

Free radicals are molecules that are missing an electron. This makes them extremely unstable, so they try to steal electrons from other molecules. Depriving other molecules of electrons makes them free radicals too, and so on it goes in a destructive chain reaction. This process is called oxidation and is very much like rusting.

Some free radicals are formed as a by-product of our normal cellular metabolism and by our immune system to fight off infections and other foreign invaders in a selective manner; others are generated by environmental factors such as pollution, radiation, cigarette smoke and horticultural chemicals. Normally antioxidants control oxidation but when too many free radicals are being produced and too few antioxidants are available then cell damage can occur. Damage from free radicals accumulates with age.

- the fatty layers of your cell membranes
- your skin's DNA
- protein — namely your collagen and elastin.

A break or alteration in your DNA can cause mutations that, over time, can lead not only cancer but also degenerative changes in your collagen and elastin fibres, making your skin prematurely prone to sagging and wrinkles. It can also force pores (which rely on these fibres to stay tight) to open and appear larger.

Free radicals can cause collagen and elastin in your dermis (the middle layer) to harden and thicken so that the collagen fibres twist and bind together in a process called cross-linking. Because the firm, wrinkle-free look of skin depends on collagen to be flexible and orderly, cross-linking causes your skin to sag and wrinkle. Plus your skin is no longer resilient enough to resist the habitual expression patterns. Free radicals can also stimulate production of collagen-digesting enzymes. Not good news for your skin's bounce! It's the excessive production of free radicals that encourages skin damage and accelerates ageing.

Antioxidants — anti-age, anti-disease

A study published in *Clinical and Experimental Dermatology* found that consuming increased levels of antioxidants in the form of fruits and vegetables has a protective effect against oxidative stress.[15] This is because the phytonutrients in fruits and vegetables contain some of the most powerful anti-oxidant systems to fight these free radicals.

Women and antioxidants

Women need all the antioxidants they can get. According to research at the University of California in Berkeley, women experience more oxidative damage than men, and more free-radical damage that can contribute to premature ageing. Researcher Gladys Block, Professor of Epidemiology and Public Health Nutrition at Berkeley, speculates that higher levels of body fat in women may be a source of these free radicals. Poor skin tone can be a sign of an antioxidant deficiency.

To see how antioxidants work, try this: Cut an apple in half. Dip one half in lemon juice. Leave the other half the way it is. Wait for an hour. You'll notice that half of the apple has turned brown — the result of free radical damage caused by contact with the oxygen in the air. The other half of the apple — the part dipped in lemon juice — will still be crisp and white. Why the difference? Lemon juice contains vitamin C, which acts as an antioxidant. So coating the apple with lemon juice effectively creates a shield against free radical damage.

The pigments that give fruits and vegetables their colour are potent phytonutrient antioxidants. Vegetables or fruits that are very bright or rich in colour — such as deep-green vegetables like spinach or bright blueberries — are packed with phytonutrient antioxidant systems such as polyphenols. Polyphenols act as potent scavengers of free radicals throughout your body, including within your skin.

Other phytonutrients such as the carotenoids and flavonoids, found in a wide variety of fruits and vegetables, are vital for strengthening your cell membranes and protecting collagen. Additionally, flavonoids protect your blood vessels and strengthen the tiny capillaries that deliver oxygen and essential nutrients to all cells. Strong cell membranes help regenerate and protect the integrity of your skin and, in doing so, can help slow ageing. Flavonoids also help to raise levels of the antioxidant molecule glutathione, and they help to keep inflammation in check. Scientists agree that the best way to get the benefits from the different phytonutrients is by eating a wide variety of fruits and vegetables.

It's worth noting that some fruits and vegetables are significantly richer in antioxidants than others. Listed on page 27 are the top twenty antioxidant-rich fruit and vegetables according to a scale called the ORAC, or Oxygen Radical Absorbance Capacity, scale. The ORAC scale was developed by researchers at Tuft's University in the United States to measure the total antioxidant power of fruits and vegetables and other plant foods such as nuts, grains and legumes. The higher the ORAC score, the more capable that particular food is of neutralising free radicals and thereby helping to slow the ageing process.

The Top 20 Antioxidant Foods according to the ORAC Scale[16]

TOP TEN FRUITS	TOP TEN VEGETABLES
Blueberries	Artichokes
Prunes	Broccoli
Blackberries	Red cabbage
Raspberries	Red (Pontiac) potatoes
Strawberries	Yellow onions
Red delicious apples	Asparagus
Granny Smith apples	Yellow, orange or red capsicums
Cherries	Beetroot
Plums	Spinach
Gala apples	Sweet potatoes

Nuts that came out top of the antioxidant list include walnuts, pecans, pistachios and hazelnuts. Dates (Deglet variety), figs and raisins were also found to be particularly rich in antioxidants. Many of the beans, including red kidney, black beans, navy and pinto, were found to be sky high in antioxidants.

You'll see that ORAC values are higher in darker coloured fruits and vegetables than in lighter ones. Go for spinach over celery, blueberries over bananas. Think colour! Numerous studies have shown that eating plenty of high-ORAC foods such as spinach and blueberries raises the antioxidant levels in of human blood by a whopping 10 to 25 per cent! Try to eat lots of deep, intense and vibrantly coloured fruits and vegetables each day. A baby spinach salad, vine-ripened tomatoes, green and red capsicums, broccoli florets, Spanish

Simple ways to boost your phytonutrient antioxidant intake

BREAKFAST

Add fresh strawberries, raspberries, blueberries, or prunes to natural yoghurt. Make a compote of dried prunes, apricots, and peaches pre-soaked in mineral water and sprinkled with flaked almonds or pecans.

LUNCH AND DINNER

Try gazpacho soup made with fresh tomatoes, green and red capsicums, onions, and cucumber with lemon juice. Eat a green salad of young spinach leaves, avocado, broccoli florets and green capsicums. Add artichoke hearts. Make a Greek salad with tomatoes, red and green capsicums, cucumber and onion.

DESSERT

Indulge in pawpaw with lime juice, fruit salad with mango, rockmelon and red grapes. Try a mix of strawberries, raspberries, blackberries and red and black currants.

DRINKS

Sip fresh fruit and vegetable juices; carrot, mango and orange juices are great for the skin. Fresh strawberry and raspberry smoothies make a delicious alternative.

SNACKS

Mixed unsalted nuts, sunflower and pumpkin seeds, raisins, carrots and fresh cherries.

onion and grated carrot will give you the benefits of a broad spectrum of age-defying antioxidants to protect your skin and to help slow the ageing process naturally.

 TIP

To optimise the phytonutrient content of foods, buy fruits and vegetables in season; limit peeling, as some phytonutrients are concentrated in the skin; and steam to cook, using minimal liquid to preserve water-soluble phytonutrients.

Whether you eat your fruit and vegetables fresh, frozen, processed or cooked can also affect its antioxidant potency — for good and bad. For example, blueberries are best eaten fresh rather than cooked in a pie. On the other hand, gently cooking tomatoes raises their antioxidant power.

As a bonus, phytonutrients found in fresh fruits and vegetables defend your body not only against premature ageing but also against genetic mutations that can lead to diseases like cancer and diabetes. In the same way that a coat of paint stops iron from rusting, antioxidants keep free radicals from eating away at collagen and elastin in your skin. So the more antioxidants you have floating around your bloodstream from the fruit and vegetables you've eaten, the more disease protection you'll have, and the healthier you and your skin will be. You'll also be less vulnerable to chronic degenerative disease and ageing. Your skin will look gorgeous and your body will be glowing on the inside too!

Optimise your pH balance

Now let's look more closely at the role of fruits and vegetables in creating an optimal pH state (the measure of acidity relative to alkalinity) in the body. The acid–alkaline balance is an important factor in the health and functioning of your body, and a good acid–alkaline regulation is vital for gorgeous skin. But the average Western diet is largely acid forming — high in protein, processed foods, refined sugars and starches. An acidic pH can also result from emotional stress, toxic overload, and/or immune reactions, or any process that deprives your cells of oxygen and other nutrients — in short, from living today!

Too much acidity in your body can reduce your ability to absorb minerals and other nutrients, decrease energy production in your cells, decrease your ability to repair damaged cells and detoxify heavy metals, and it can make you more susceptible to fatigue and illness. Highly acidic diets also result in the excretion of your important beauty minerals such as calcium, magnesium and zinc.

An acidic system makes it so much more difficult to achieve your goal of gorgeous skin. Your body tries to compensate for the acidic pH by 'stealing' your stores of alkaline minerals. And if your diet doesn't contain enough minerals to compensate, acid can build up in your cells. The right food can actually change the course of your biochemistry. The bottom line is that fresh fruits and vegetables

TIP

Choose fruits and vegetables that are low on the glycaemic index (GI).

Low-GI fruits and vegetables release a steady stream of glucose into your bloodstream so you won't get that age-accelerating spike of insulin. Asparagus, beans, broccoli, cabbage, blueberries, peaches, pears, spinach and most non-starchy vegetables are all low-GI foods. (For details of the glycaemic index, see page 53.)

create an optimal alkaline state, while animal products, processed starches and sugars create acids and reduce oxygen and vitality.

Supercharge your servings

It's one thing to know that you need to eat lots of fruits and vegetables. But you just can't eat too many of these foods for gorgeous skin. And unless you're consuming the recommended five to nine servings of fresh fruit and vegies every day, you're probably fighting a losing battle against the daily onslaught of free radicals. For extra protection, I recommend adding a whole-food fruit and vegetable supplement to your diet on top of the Gorgeous Skin supplements detailed in Chapter 4. Opt for one that contains a full spectrum of concentrated natural phytonutrients, vitamins, minerals and antioxidants, as they exist in whole food form such as Juice Plus+ or other similar products. (See Resources, page 304, for further information.)

Another way of optimising the performance of what you eat is to go organic. The Gorgeous Skin program advocates organically grown foods wherever possible. Organic fruits and vegetables are pesticide-free and are grown in healthy soil that hasn't been con-taminated by lots of nasty chemicals such as pesticides, herbicides, chemical fertilisers, GM organisms and additives. Each of these chem-icals can contribute to toxic overload, put pressure on your liver, and encourage free-radical damage. And research shows that organics tend to have much higher nutritional values.

According to Dr Jeffery Bland, author of the *20-Day Rejuvenation Diet*, 'exposure to toxic chemicals like pesticides increases the level of oxidative stress on the body'.[17] Upwards of a thousand different chemicals are routinely applied to crops! Essentially, these chemicals increase your body's free-radical load. Exposure to various chemicals and pesticides also depletes your body's antioxidant nutrients — including glutathione, one of your main detoxifying nutrients, which among other things helps trap free radicals in your liver to prevent further damage.

Studies show that levels of nutrients are consistently higher in organic fruit and vegetables than in non-organic produce.[18] A study published in 2001 in the US *Journal of Alternative and Complementary Medicine* found that organically-grown produce was on average twenty to thirty per cent higher in a wide variety of different vitamins and minerals.[19] New research has also shown that organics have much higher levels of antioxidants too. Crops that are stressed by insects naturally produce polyphenolic (phytonutrient) compounds, which are potent antioxidants.[20] But crops that are treated with pesticides don't need the natural protection of these beneficial polyphenolics, so they produce less of these compounds. So you get a double benefit when crops aren't sprayed with pesticides: better nutrition (higher levels of nutrients and antioxidants) and no residue from chemical pesticides. Also, due to intensive farming methods, the soil in which non-organic produce is grown is often depleted of minerals, which ultimately means that fewer nutrients reach the food. Plus, organic fruit and vegetables are so much tastier too.

By eating organics you also won't be consuming any genetically modified (GM) organisms, as they are outlawed in the production of organic food. Independent research conducted on GM foods has found evidence of the damaging effects of GM foods to the gut lining in humans. Reports from these studies caution that until GM crops and food products are properly tested, people are wise to avoid eating GM food.[21] Another reason to go organic is that many of the pesticides and other chemicals used in the spraying process

TIP

If you can't get hold of organically grown fruit and vegetables, then wash the standard ones well in a hydrogen-peroxide solution to help remove the chemicals. This will also keep your food fresher longer.

Mix 1 cup of 3 per cent hydrogen peroxide (found at your supermarket or chemist) with 8 litres of water (purified water is best). Soak thin-skinned fruits and leafy vegetables for fifteen minutes and thick-skinned fruits and vegetables for thirty minutes. Rinse well and let stand in purified water for at least ten minutes. Drain and dry well before eating.

are 'xenoestrogens'. These are compounds that mimic the effect of oestrogen in the body in not-so-fabulous ways. There have been numerous links made between xenoestrogens and a variety of cancers, including breast cancer.[22]

And if you're thinking that organic food is too hard to come by, things have changed a lot over the past few years. There was a time when organics were available only in health-food stores. But, thanks to public demand, you can now find organic fruits and vegetables and other products in most supermarkets, including the major chains. And even the prices are coming down, with more growers entering the market.

Face fats

You may be surprised to know that fat is actually a very close runner-up to fruits and vegetables in terms of its nutritional importance for your skin. In fact, depriving yourself of fat can cause all sorts of skin problems, along with hair loss and hormonal imbalances. If you're getting fewer than 20 grams of fat a day (roughly 2 tablespoons of oil), your skin may not be able to lubricate itself and your body may not absorb enough vitamin A, which your skin needs to prevent premature ageing and to look its absolute best.

Without fat you also won't absorb the beneficial phytonutrients like carotenoids or lycopene that are so great for your skin. A study published in the *Journal of the American College of Nutrition* found that a group of participants who ate a salad with a non-fat dressing had no absorption of carotenoids![23] In fact, after eating the salad with a fat-free dressing, participants turned in blood tests showing negligible levels of alpha-carotene, beta-carotene and lycopene in all subjects. And a substantially greater absorption of carotenoids was observed when salads were consumed with full-fat rather than reduced-fat salad dressing. So forget going fat-free!

The key is to eat the right kind of fats, and in the right balance. For soft, supple, and lustrous skin, it's absolutely essential that you eat enough 'good' fat every day. As you'll discover, even though all fats, gram for gram, contain the same number of kilojoules, they certainly aren't all equal as far as your health (and therefore your skin) is concerned.

The following fats will all do your skin good:
- Olive oil — extra-virgin, cold-pressed
- Flaxseed oil — organic, cold-pressed (but *never* heated)
- Walnut oil — organic, cold-pressed
- Pumpkin seed oil — organic, cold-pressed
- Coconut oil — virgin, cold-pressed
- Mustard seed oil
- Avocado oil
- Soy oil — organic
- Macadamia nut oil — cold-pressed
- Canola oil — make sure it's cold pressed, and preferably organic as most canola oil, along with grapeseed oil, is obtained through chemical extraction (as opposed to mechanical pressing), which may leave trace solvents in the oils.

From a beauty point of view, 'good' fats:
- stimulate collagen synthesis
- help keep skin moist and supple
- improve blood flow and nutrient delivery to your cells
- aid absorption of your beauty vitamins A, D, E and K and phytonutrients like the carotenoids, lycopene and lutein

- help produce and regulate hormones
- fend off eczema, psoriasis, dryness and hair loss
- assist in detoxing
- reduce inflammation — of skin, among other things.

Good fat, bad fat

Fats are made up of fatty acids, and fatty acids come as three types: saturated, monounsaturated or polyunsaturated. Each type is metabolised and used differently by the body; for good health we need to supply our bodies with the right amount of each.

Saturated fatty acids are easy to recognise: they're solid at room temperature. Saturated fats are found in foods such as butter, palm oils, beef, chicken and pork fat, and full-fat dairy products such as cheese and ice-cream. With the exception of coconut oil, and small amounts of organic butter, the saturated fats aren't the best for your skin, although they can have other health benefits.

Monounsaturated fatty acids are liquid at room temperature. They are found in foods such as olive oil, canola oil, cashews, macadamia nuts, avocados and oily, cold-water fish such as swordfish, mackerel and salmon.

Take note of the monounsaturates because research has shown that eating foods high in monounsaturated fatty acids can lessen the impact of wrinkles!

Coconut comes out of the closet

The new buzz in the 'fat' world is coconut oil. Yes, it's a saturated fat and we've all been told for years that saturated fats bump up cholesterol levels and clog arteries. But there are three different types of saturated fats, and coconuts contain the healthiest type, with medium-chain fatty acids (MCFAs) that will actually help you lose weight while keeping you healthy. Whereas other fats are stored in the body's cells, the MCFAs in coconut oil are sent directly to the liver where they are immediately converted into energy. So when you eat coconut and coconut oil your body uses the food immediately for energy rather than storing it as body fat! Plus, in addition to tasting and smelling great, coconut oil is an amazing fat for your skin — internally and externally.

Polyunsaturated fatty acids are similar to monounsaturated fatty acids in that they're also liquid at room temperature but they have a slightly different molecular structure. Polyunsaturated fatty acids are found mostly in foods such as flax seeds, walnuts and oily cold-water fish, as well as in safflower, sunflower and corn oils. Polyunsaturated fatty acids are also known as the essential fatty acids, or EFAs, and are divided into two major classes: Omega-6 and Omega-3 fatty acids. These are the 'good oils', but (as you'll see) only if taken in the right proportions.

Fabulous flaxseed ... and other good oils

Flaxseed oil contains all of the important essential fatty acids for a beautiful complexion and great health. It's also a wonderful wrinkle softener and moisturises the skin from the inside. But its essential fatty acids are extremely sensitive to heat and are quickly destroyed in the cooking process, so it should always be refrigerated and never be used in cooking. Other good oils are coconut, avocado and macadamia, along with walnut, mustard seed and pumpkin oil (but never heat these last three).

Essential Fatty Acids (EFAs) — the best fats

EFAs are like the team leaders in your body's work force. They're important building blocks for cell membranes; when cell membranes are healthy, they transport nutrients efficiently, giving your skin a great glow. A balanced and sufficient intake of EFAs can also help you burn body fat, give you energy and encourage your skin to hold water, making it smooth and youthful. EFAs are also vital for your brain and nerve cells.

Your body can make all the fat it needs, except for two essential fatty acids: linoleic acid (LA) and alpha-linolenic acid (ALA). It's vital that you get these fatty acids through your diet or through a regular intake of supplements; that's why they're known as 'essential'. LA is the head of the Omega-6 family of fats and ALA is the head of the Omega-3 family. These two EFAs are found naturally in fresh food such as fish, wild game, seeds and nuts, and green leafy vegetables.

OMEGA-6	OMEGA-3
Sunflower oil	Fish and fish oils
Corn oil	Canola oil
Safflower oil	Flax seeds & flaxseed oil
Cottonseed oil	Walnuts & walnut oil
Soybean oil (unless it's cold pressed, unrefined and not hydrogenated)	Soybeans and unrefined, unhydrogenated soybean oil
Evening primrose oil	Mustard seed oil and mustard seeds
Borage oil	Dark-green leafy vegetables

From a beauty point of view, essential fatty acids:
- build strong cell walls for beautiful, well-hydrated skin
- ensure insulin sensitivity and good blood glucose (sugar) control
- reduce excessive inflammation
- maintain cellular hydration.

The danger of inflammation

Inflammation is one indicator of free radical damage and it can accelerate ageing like nobody's business! Inflammation can be both visible and invisible. Sunburn is a visible type of inflammation; it's the result of your body defending itself against the trauma of UV rays. High levels of hormones such as insulin (due to high blood sugar levels) and your stress hormone cortisol can cause the 'silent' type of inflammation. You can't see silent inflammation and you can't feel it; it occurs deep in your cells and it can activate certain molecules (called transcription factors), which in turn can lead to more inflammation and accelerate the ageing process. Scientists are now learning that inflammation also plays a critical role in the development of many of the diseases of ageing such as diabetes, heart disease, and cancer.

A deficiency or imbalance in essential fatty acids can age skin before its time. From a structural perspective, even though the *stratum corneum* (the very outer layer of your epidermis) is composed of dead cells, its ability to form a tight junction is critical for stopping the skin from losing water. The first sign of an essential fatty acid deficiency is the breakdown of this barrier, resulting in dry, flaking skin, psoriasis, eczema or chronic skin problems.

In the body, Omega-3 and Omega-6 fatty acids are converted into hormone-like substances called eicosanoids. Eicosanoids can have a profound influence on your health and beauty. Eicosanoids produced from Omega-3 and Omega-6 fatty acids have opposite functions. Omega-3s decrease inflammation; on the other hand too many Omega-6s can increase inflammation. The fats you eat make up your cell walls, and for optimum health and beauty you need really flexible cell walls. But when you eat too many of the highly refined Omega-6 fats, and other 'bad' skin fats including the truly unhealthy trans fatty acids — or trans fats (which appear on the ingredient list as 'hydrogenated' or 'partially hydrogenated' vegetable oils and they're also found in fried foods and margarine; see pages 142–3), your cell walls can become stiff and inflexible which causes myriad problems. This makes it all the more difficult for nutrients to pass through to feed your cells, circulation can become sluggish, and ultimately this can lead to greasy pores, acne and dry flaky skin. Stiff cells walls also mean that cells can become less responsive to messages from your hormones and other important molecules. Seriously bad news for your skin. So you can influence your health and beauty simply by choosing one type of fatty acid over another.

It's all about balance: increase the 3s while decreasing the 6s! Balancing Omega-3 and Omega-6 EFAs is absolutely vital for your goal of gorgeous skin. When these two essential fatty acids are balanced, you have a much lower risk of inflammation and other diseases as well. The big problem these days is that our diets are overloaded with Omega-6 fatty acids and are often deficient in Omega-3s. The optimal ratio of Omega-6 to Omega-3 for your health and therefore skin is 4:1 or 3:1. But these days, thanks to our diets and lifestyles, the ratio hovers somewhere around 14:1 to 20:1, which is bad news for skin.

Virtually all processed and take-away food is loaded with Omega-6 oils. Regular refined vegetable oils like sunflower, safflower and corn oil found in supermarkets are also full of Omega-6 oils. Even if you opt for a salad, most dressings are made with cheap, refined oils that are high in Omega-6 fatty acids. The same goes for most inexpensive take-away foods. Too many of these Omega-6 oils — especially the less expensive, highly refined ones — can provoke and stimulate inflammation and cause a whole host of other problems, including less than gorgeous skin. (Chapter 6 contains more detailed information about the effects of excessive Omega-6 oils.)

But Omega-6 fatty acids are not all bad for your skin. In the right form and balance, Omega-6s such as supplementary evening primrose oil (EPO) and borage seed oil can give your skin a real beauty boost. But it's the Omega-3 fatty acids that are the real stars for your skin. The Omega-3 family of fatty acids supplies the building blocks of a variety of powerful anti-inflammatory substances. The Omega-3s also help build strong cell walls for beautiful, well-hydrated skin and in doing so can make your skin smoother, softer and more radiant. So the

 TIP

Try to avoid commercial salad dressings. Make your own. Mix cold-pressed virgin olive oil, fresh lemon juice or balsamic vinegar, and fresh herbs.

To increase your Omega-3 intake:

- grind whole flaxseeds in a coffee grinder and sprinkle over fresh fruit
- throw a handful of walnuts into a green leafy salad
- add a tablespoon of flaxseed oil to your morning smoothie
- eat oily, cold-water fish like salmon, mackerel or tuna at least three times a week.

bottom line is: too many Omega-6 oils can cause inflammation and premature ageing, whereas Omega-3s can be your skin's best friend. But in the right balance, these two EFAs will make your skin glow and your hair shine.

Fat phobics take note: EFAs will not make you fat. In fact, they can have the opposite effect. In the right balance, EFAs increase your metabolic rate so that more of your stored fat can be burned as energy. They increase your cell's sensitivity to insulin, allowing your body to do its job of regulating blood sugar. EFAs can also help it break down and eliminate cholesterol and bad fats from your system, and even help to smooth and tone problem areas where cellulite might lurk.

Olive oil — the odd one out

One oil that is highly beneficial to the skin is neither an Omega-3 nor an Omega-6 EFA, but an Omega-9 — and that's olive oil. Long regarded as the 'beauty oil', olive oil is rich in mono-unsaturated fats — along with avocado, canola oil and most nuts — and in vitamins A, B1, B2, C, D, E, K and iron. It also contains lots of fabulous phytonutrients such as the flavones.

 TIP

As olive oil is more resistant to the effects of heat and light than polyunsaturated oils, it's more stable and better for cooking. Use cold-pressed extra-virgin olive oil in your salads and even for wok-frying foods. (Virgin olive oils are always unrefined.) If you're after a different taste, cold-pressed macadamia nut oil is a good substitute for olive oil. Macadamia nut oil is rich in anti-inflammatory oleic acid, the same Omega-9 fat found in olive oil. It also has a high smoke point, so you can cook with it at higher temperatures than you can with olive oil. Coconut oil is also good for cooking at high temperatures as it's very stable.

Your body's cells incorporate the valuable fats from olive oil, making arteries more supple and skin more lustrous. Research shows that people who consume the most olive oil — along with fish, nuts, and fresh fruits and vegetables — have the least skin wrinkling.[24]

As you start eating more of the skin-friendly fats and swapping

TIP

Purchase oils in small quantities, keep them refrigerated, and toss out any unused oils after three months. All oils — especially flaxseed — gradually oxidise or turn rancid, the result of age as well as exposure to light and air. Rancid oils contain a fiesta of free radicals and can harm your health.

bad fats for good fats, you'll be amazed at the difference in your skin. Hard and dry skin, greasy pores, pimples, bumps and acne will begin to disappear. Your skin will feel velvety, smooth and lovely to touch. As an added bonus, you'll also get an enhanced feeling of wellbeing. For optimum benefit, try to include two to four tablespoons of the good fats each day. When your skin is buttery smooth, reduce your intake to two tablespoons per day.

Protein power

It wasn't that long ago that we were told to load up on carbohydrates and limit our protein and fat, but the Atkins and South Beach diets have changed all of that. We now know that high-protein diets balance insulin levels and help shed weight. But protein is also absolutely essential for gorgeous skin. In fact, protein is equated with beauty because your hair, skin and nails are about ninety-eight per cent protein! Ample protein staves off the visible signs of ageing, whereas a deficiency can result in weak nails, premature ageing, hair loss, and even droopy facial muscles.

Protein is absolutely essential for a whole host of other reasons too: it helps repair the damage done to your body's cells by free radicals, helps make the powerhouse antioxidant glutathione, creates vital enzymes to zap toxins, maintains energy levels and helps keep your blood sugar levels in balance by supporting your adrenal glands, pancreas and liver.

Having low protein levels increases your desire for carbohydrates, like sugar, which contributes to a rise in insulin levels. High insulin levels spell disaster for your skin. In fact, a lack of adequate protein prevents cellular repair, which can put you on a fast track to ageing.

And since your body can't store protein, it's essential that you get adequate amounts daily. The best sources of protein for luminous, radiant skin are from fish, free-range poultry, wild game, unprocessed soy, micro-filtered whey and organic eggs.

It is now clear that high-carbohydrate diets inflate the appetite and foster type 2 diabetes, but eating healthily is certainly not just about protein and fat. You can have your carbohydrates and eat them too! You just have to know how to chose them. It's the refined carbohydrates that are the baddies, as they can trigger a toxic cascade by causing extreme surges in blood sugar and insulin, which in turn can contribute to weight gain, inflammation and eventually accelerated ageing. The trick is to choose carbohydrates with a low GI (see table page 53). Dr Atkins certainly deserves credit for publicising the perils of refined carbs, but the centrepiece of the original Atkins diet — eating unlimited amounts of beef, sausage, butter and cheese — is a bad idea, whether you're on the gorgeous skin program or not. Although it can be hugely successful for weight loss, it's not a prescription for optimal health and beauty.

Get hooked on fish

Asian people, whose diets are high in fish, are known for their beautiful complexion. This is because gorgeous skin needs the good fats in fish, and lots of them. Fish and most other seafoods contain a powerhouse of the beauty-boosting Omega-3 EFAs. Salmon, sardines, tuna, mackerel, snapper and cod are loaded with Omega-3 EFAs, along with dimethylaminoethanol, or DMAE for short. DMAE is a compound found in high levels in anchovies, wild salmon, and sardines, and small amounts of it are also naturally produced in the human brain. DMAE increases tone in the skin and helps protect the integrity of cell membranes.

If you think you eat enough fish and seafood, think again! Most

Go fatty

Fatty seafood has more benefits than lean seafood. Lean seafoods, including cod, flounder, crab and prawns, have about one-twentieth of the Omega-3 EFAs that are in oily fish. Fish fingers and deep-fried fish contain even less. And even though some fish contains ten times more fat than other fish, it's still lean relative to poultry and meat. Fish has all the protein of beef, and less than half the fat.

of us aren't getting enough Omega-3 fatty acids to meet the daily dietary recommendations and one indicator of this is our weekly fish consumption. Unless you eat fatty fish two or more times a week, or take Omega-3 supplements, you're likely to be deficient in both docosahexaenoic acid (DHA) and eicosapentaenoic acid (EPA), which are so fabulous for your skin. All fish contain EPA and DHA; however-er, the quantities vary among species and within a species according to environmental variables such as diet and whether the fish are wild or farm raised. If you can't stand seafood, 2000 milligrams of a fish-oil supplement has the same amount of healthy fats as a 150 gram serving of salmon. Don't worry: it doesn't taste fishy!

 TIP

When cooking fish, stick to methods such as baking, poaching, steaming and grilling. Frying fish destroys the beneficial fatty acids and creates free radicals.

How safe is your salmon?

Salmon is packed with Omega-3 fatty acids, CoQ10, DMAE and protein — all sensational skin nutrients. But there's a catch, as this generally applies to wild salmon. Most of the salmon and trout available today comes not from the sea but from fish farms and unfortunately farmed fish doesn't have as many of the health benefits of wild fish.

Farmed salmon are raised in crowded net pens. They're fattened with soybean pellets and other cereal-based chow. This changes their essential fatty acid ratio, making them higher in saturated fat and linoleic acid (an Omega-6 fatty acid), and lower in the beneficial

Mercury mayhem

From time to time the media raises issues about mercury levels in fish. But are these concerns justified? As with many discussions about trace levels of toxins, the one involving mercury in seafood stems from failing to realise that it is the dose that makes it poisonous.

It is true that mercury is toxic, and reports of its tragic effects in humans were reported back in the 1950s near Minamata Bay, Japan. There, residents had extremely high exposure to seafood from waters where tonnes of mercury had been released. However, numerous studies of less extreme circumstances, including a nine-year-long study of children with high prenatal exposure to mercury, have indicated that low levels of mercury do not cause harm in humans. And a study published in *The Lancet* in May 2003 found no evidence that low levels of mercury in seafood had harmful effects on women or children.[25] This research was conducted in the Seychelles islands where the fish contain the same levels of mercury as fish consumed in Australia and the United States. But more importantly the Seychellians eat on average 12 fish meals per week, almost 10 times the amount of fish we do!

Mercury gets into water primarily through solid-waste incinerators, mines and power plants. Algae absorbs the mercury, tiny zooplankton animals eat the algae, small fish eat the zooplankton, and from there the mercury works up through the aquatic food chain, with the large, deep-ocean fish at the top of the chain carrying the highest mercury concentration.

According to Food Standards Australia and New Zealand (FSANZ) we should continue eating several serves of fish and seafood per week but avoid fish high in mercury, such as shark, swordfish, king mackerel and marlin. These are long-lived predatory fish that accumulate mercury in the form of methyl mercury. Fish previously classed as high in mercury but now off the high-mercury list are ray, gemfish, ling and southern bluefin tuna. Pregnant women, women planning pregnancy and children up to six years old are also advised to restrict consumption of orange roughy (sea perch) and catfish. Nursing mothers are advised that, if they want to be cautious, they should also follow the advice for pregnant women.

My advice to everyone else is: cut back on eating deep-ocean fish like swordfish too often, and vary your fish as much as possible, because the benefits of these valuable essential fats far outweigh the risks.

Omega-3 fatty acids. They're also fed antibiotics to ward off myriad diseases that are uncommon in wild salmon, and they're likely to be exposed to heavy doses of unhealthy hormones and pesticides, not to mention their own nitrogenous fish waste.

Wild salmon eat creatures like shrimp and krill, which contain chemicals that make salmon pink. Farm-raised salmon don't eat these forms of sea life, so they're artificially coloured to make them look like wild salmon. The colours that are added to the salmon's feed are canthaxanthin and astaxanthin, which are produced both naturally and synthetically. This information is particularly important for people with sensitivity to food dyes. Also, farmed salmon has been found to contain toxic chemicals, including PCBs, other dioxins and various pesticide residues. All are known or suspected causes of cancer, neurological problems, immune suppression and/or hormonal disruption.

My advice is: Eat farmed salmon only occasionally, and where possible seek out wild salmon. Canned salmon is generally wild. The same Omega-3 fatty acids found in salmon can be obtained from sardines and mackerel, as well as from walnuts and flax seeds.

Lean poultry

Chicken, wild game, eggs and turkey are all great sources of protein for your skin. Just be sure to buy organic or free-range, as conventionally raised poultry tends to be loaded with antibiotics and hormones, which can wreak havoc on your hormones and create skin problems. Also, grill or bake poultry, but avoid frying at all costs.

Sensational soy

Whole, unprocessed soy foods are an excellent source of high-quality digestible protein. In fact, soy is the only plant food that is a complete protein, meaning that it contains all the essential amino acids that the body can't produce. It's also high in antioxidants, vitamins, minerals and protective phytonutrients called soy isoflavones. Each of these isoflavones has unique benefits, but together they act synergistically; that's why it's far better to consume soy in whole form. (See Chapter 3 for its other great health and skin benefits.)

Whole soy comes in the following forms:

- tempeh
- miso
- tofu
- soy milk
- textured vegetable protein (also known as TVP — available at selected health food shops).

 TIP

Opt for non-genetically modified (non-GMO) soy, preferably organic. These days, almost 95 per cent of soybeans come from GMO seeds.

Micro-filtered whey

Micro-filtered whey is another excellent source of protein for gorgeous skin. It boosts cell renewal, new tissue growth and lean muscle mass. It improves skin by increasing levels of glutathione, the age-retarding antioxidant extraordinaire, which is believed to improve the quality of collagen in connective tissue and skin. There is also evidence that it may help prevent cross-linking of collagen that comes with ageing.

 TIP

For a real beauty boost make a quick morning shake with 20 to 30 grams of micro-filtered whey protein powder, a teaspoon of flaxseed oil, an apple, a pear or a handful of berries, and blend with a few ice cubes and filtered water.

Great grains

Think whole grain for beautiful skin. Grains are 'whole' when they include the bran, germ and the thin cellophane skin, all of which are particularly rich in the vitamins, minerals, phytonutrients, oils and proteins that will help to keep your skin firm, smooth and supple. Refined grains are stripped of the bran, skin and germ — a process that also removes the majority of fibre and nutrients but leaves behind nearly all the kilojoules! Fibre slows down the rate at which glucose is absorbed into your bloodstream, giving your body more time to process carbohydrates, leading to lower blood sugar levels, better carbohydrate metabolism, and less age-accelerating insulin. Fibre also strengthens the large intestine and helps keep elimination smooth and regular, and your body toxin-free. Whole grains are also far lower on the glycaemic index than refined grains.

Not only does the refining process remove nutrients, but it also concentrates the sugar within simple-carbohydrate foods. This can overstress your pancreas, the organ responsible for removing sugar (glucose) from your bloodstream and moving it into muscle cells to be burned as fuel. This can manifest as insulin over-secretion, causing (for a while, anyway, until it gives up) low blood sugar levels with a subsequent vicious cycle of blood sugar over-shooting and under-shooting as the body tries to auto-regulate. And in the long term it increases inflammation and accelerates ageing. So always choose the whole food, like brown rice over white. And when you buy bread, be sure to read the label! Most 'wheat' breads are refined; only true 'whole grain' breads will have any beauty and nutritive value.

The good grains are:
- brown rice
- quinoa
- kasha (available in selected health-food shops)
- buckwheat
- millet
- amaranth (available in selected health-food stores)

- wild rice
- oats
- barley.

Fibre is an important part of a healthy diet and is a must for a beautiful complexion. A fairly typical highly processed, low-fibre Western diet can lead to stagnation in the intestines and digestive tract and can eventually result in a build-up of toxicity. A toxic body equals blemishes, pimples, boils and congested-looking skin. According to Avelin Kushi, author of several macrobiotic books and wife of Michio Kushi, the world's leading authority on macrobiotics, 'when food starts stagnating in your intestines the body becomes less able to discharge excess fat and cholesterol, and these can circulate in the blood stream, eventually depositing in connective tissues, blood vessels, internal organs and your skin'.[26]

Australians typically consume about half the amount of fibre that's optimal for health and longevity. Luckily, it isn't difficult to increase your fibre intake, as most whole foods, fruits and vegetables are packed with fibre.

There are actually two types of fibre, each with a different function.

Insoluble fibre is the type that helps keep your digestive system in good working order. This natural laxative helps soften stools (making elimination easier) and speeds up the movement of waste material through the digestive system so you can avoid constipation. It also helps control and balance the pH (acidity) in the intestines. Good dietary sources include: whole grains, vegetables, fruits and dried peas and beans.

Soluble fibre has little effect on intestinal bulk, but it helps lower blood cholesterol levels and regulates blood sugar levels. Good dietary sources include: fruits, vegetables, oats, barley and dried peas and beans.

Going against the grain

Some grains contain a protein called gluten that can be problematic for a lot of unsuspecting people. Gluten is an umbrella term for forty related proteins in a handful of grains, particularly in wheat, rye and barley. Gluten is a mixed blessing. Many people — approximately one in every hundred — are allergic to gluten, causing what is known as coeliac disease. But the gluten protein may cause a number of health problems for many people who do not have an inborn sensitivity to gluten and according to Melissa Diane Smith, a nutritionist and author of *Going Against the Grain,* up to half the Western population may be sensitive to gluten without exhibiting any of the traditional symptoms of coeliac disease. Instead, gluten sensitivity may appear as immune system reactions affecting the nervous system, balance and behaviour, as well as a person's overall sense of well-being. According to Smith, a second family of grain (and legume) proteins, called lectins, may also damage the gut and interfere with nutrient absorption.[27] Additionally, according to research by Dr Loren Cordain, author of *The Paleo Diet,* lectins may play a role in rheumatoid arthritis and possibly other inflammatory auto-immune diseases.[28] So go easy on these grains and if you do suspect an intolerance to gluten, substitute for other grains like brown rice that don't contain any gluten.

Beautiful beans

The beneficial phytonutrients found in beans and legumes — such as chickpeas, kidney, black and navy beans, soybeans and lentils — make them an anti-ageing necessity. They are also filled with fibre, are low on the GI index and are packed with protein. Combine them with vegetables and herbs for delicious soups, or they can be used in salads or prepared and served as dips. They're also a wonderful source of protein for vegetarians (often combined with barley, oats or rice). Beans and lentils contain flavonoids and flavonals — the anti-inflammatory antioxidants that are so great for your skin.

Just go nuts

Nuts are packed with fats that are good for your skin, plus they're a great source of protein and micronutrients and they provide significant antioxidant benefits. Almonds and soy nuts are particularly healthy choices because of their monounsaturated fat and flavonoid content. Walnuts also pack a powerful punch of Omega-3 EFAs. Other healthy choices include hazelnuts, pistachios and pecans.

Nuts are high in kilojoules, though, so it's best not to eat more than two to three tablespoons at a time. But the essential fats found in nuts can help keep your blood sugar stable for a few hours after they've been eaten, which will curb any cravings for carbohydrates and sugar. And this, in turn, can actually promote weight loss because, when your blood sugar levels are balanced, your body can burn kilojoules from its own fat stores. Most nuts contain magnesium and zinc, too, which also help to fight sugar cravings.

Try to get your nuts raw and unsalted from stores that turn their stock over fairly frequently. You can purchase raw nuts at any good wholefood market or health-food store. Canned, salted, or packaged roasted nuts aren't recommended.

Raw nuts have a high enzyme content. But beware, as they also have high amounts of phytates or enzyme inhibitors, which should be broken down before you eat them. You can do this by soaking the nuts in salted, or plain, filtered water for six to eight hours. Then drain, place the nuts on a baking sheet, and dry on low heat in the oven. Nuts prepared this way have been 'pre-digested' and will provide a quick source of energy and the full gamut of nutrients.

Almonds

Almonds are the most nutritious of all nuts. Like all nuts, they are a concentrated source of fat, but the majority of this fat (66 per cent) is a monounsaturated fatty acid, the same as that found in olive oil. So it's a 'good' skin fat.

Almonds are an excellent source of the key beauty nutrients — vitamin E, calcium, magnesium, phosphorous and potassium — as well as fair sources of minerals, particularly manganese and zinc. They are a good source of protein and carbohydrates, providing about twenty-six grams of each per cup. Almonds are also rich in the amino acid arginine (arginine is also found in other nuts and should be avoided if you have an active herpes infection, as it stimulates the herpes virus replication). Arginine is a natural vasodilator, which promotes increased blood flow by relaxing your blood vessels. Great news for skin!

Glutamic acid, another amino acid, is particularly plentiful in almonds. Glutamic acid is part of the antioxidant glutathione and helps with your body's detoxification. Almonds (and peanuts) also contain something called sphingolipids (these are fats that make up part of your cell membranes). At this stage there's no known nutritional requirement for these lipids, but they seem to play an important role in cell membrane structure and function. Plus the skin of almonds contains a number of polyphenols, many of which have significant free-radical fighting properties.

Walnuts

Walnuts are versatile and nutritious, containing high amounts of minerals. They are unique among nuts, as they're actually one of the few rich sources of plant-derived Omega-3 fatty acids (along with flax seeds and flaxseed oil). Being rich in Omega-3 fatty acids, they can help moisturise your skin internally and give it a healthy glow.

They're also rich in plant sterols (plant sterols can play a significant role in lowering cholesterol levels) and polyphenols (also found in red wine) plus they're a great source of fibre and protein, and they also provide magnesium, copper, folate and vitamin E.

It's their high Omega-3 content that requires walnuts and walnut oil to be handled with care. The Omega-3 fatty acids in walnuts are highly polyunsaturated which means they are very susceptible to heat, light and rancidity. Walnuts should be stored in the refrigerator. Walnut oil adds a wonderful flavour to salad dressings, but should also be refrigerated and must never be used for cooking.

Macadamia nuts

What makes macadamia nuts different from other nuts is their unusual fatty acid profile. They are about 80 per cent fat, but the majority is made up of stable monounsaturates, with smaller amounts of saturates and an even smaller but equal ratio of Omega-3 and Omega-6 fatty acids. They are also rich in minerals like copper, iron, magnesium, calcium, potassium and zinc.

Good carbohydrates

Just like fats, there are good and bad carbohydrates. Carbohydrates that break down quickly during digestion are the 'bad' carbohydrates, while carbohydrates that break down slowly, releasing glucose gradually into the blood stream, are 'good' carbohydrates. A specific index, called the glycaemic index (or GI for short), is used to measure how quickly a food raises our blood sugar levels after we eat it. Bad carbohydrates rate highest on the GI and good ones rate lowest.

Some examples of high-GI foods are: fat-free tofu ice-cream, rice cakes, white bread, bagels and baked potatoes. When foods are puffed, like rice cakes, their GI is so high (higher than that of table sugar) that they skyrocket off the chart. Examples of low-GI foods include: asparagus, beans, broccoli, blueberries, cabbage, rockmelon, peaches, pears, spinach and most non-starchy vegetables. Not only are these foods low on the glycaemic index, but they are also treasure troves of vitamins, minerals, enzymes, antioxidants and phytonutrients.

The reason high-GI foods are bad for your skin is that they increase the output of insulin — your anti-ageing arch enemy — and its equally notorious partner in crime, the stress hormone cortisol. A high level of insulin pushes your cellular metabolism into producing inflammatory chemicals and encourages your body to store fat. By stimulating the inflammatory chemicals in your body, you can kick-start the ageing process, and that's bad news for skin. The low-GI foods, by contrast, don't cause your blood sugar to rise to unhealthy levels. (For instance, the glycaemic effect of a wholegrain rye bread is 32 per cent less than the equivalent amount of white bread.) These foods should make up the majority of your carbohydrate intake, so that you avoid 'youth-stealing' spikes in your blood sugar level.

The GI scale is measured from 1 to 100, with glucose being given a score of 100. Foods are then measured against the speed of glucose and given a grade. Foods with a score of 0 to 50 are considered low GI, while foods with a score of 50 to 70 are considered moderate GI and those above 70 are rated as high GI.

Curb the bad carbs

As a result of their unique biochemistry, women have less of the 'feel-good' brain chemical serotonin than men do and levels of serotonin drop even lower during menstrual cycles. In order to raise levels of this feel-good chemical, women tend to crave high-GI foods (such as bread, biscuits, sweets and chocolate) to boost levels of serotonin.

These types of carbohydrates will certainly raise serotonin levels and make you feel good for a while, but once blood sugar levels go up and an insulin response occurs, serotonin levels will crash again.

This continual carb craving can lead to weight gain, depression and wrinkles! So go low GI and make sure you add a little protein and essential fats to each meal. This will keep off the kilos and keep your mood elevated!

The Glycaemic Index of Common Foods

FOOD	RATING	FOOD	RATING	FOOD	RATING
Glucose	100	White rice	72	Corn	59
Baked potato	98	Bagels	72	Potato chips	51
French baguette	95	White bread	69	Spaghetti	50
Gluten-free bread	95	Mars Bar	68	Oatmeal	49
Instant rice	90	Sponge cake	67	Apple	39
Honey	87	Croissant	67	Tomato	38
Cornflakes	82	Shredded wheat	67	Yoghurt	36
Pretzels	82	Brown rice	66	Whole milk	34
Doughnuts	76	Raisins	64	Skim milk	32
Waffles	76	Beetroots	64	Peanuts	13
Corn chips	73	Bananas	39		

Foods with a low GI (less than 50)

FOOD	RATING	FOOD	RATING
Vegetables		**Cereal grains**	
Spinach	20	Rye kernels	47
Asparagus	15	Barley, pearled	36
Red capsicum	15	**Fruit**	
Broccoli	14	Pineapple — canned,	48
Mushrooms	10	unsweetened	
Legumes		Grapes	45
Chickpeas, dried	47	Apple	39 (average)
Kidney beans, dried	43	Pear	34
Lima beans	36	Peach	29
Black-eyed peas	33	Grapefruit	26
Lentils	28 (average)	Plums	25
Soybeans, dried	20	**Fructose**	25

If you consume foods with a score of between 50 and 70, try to combine them with a low-rating carbohydrate to even out the overall score. For example, bananas have a high score, whereas oats and skimmed milk have a low score. If you combined all three at your breakfast you would bring down the overall score and still be able to enjoy the odd banana for its flavour and nutritional value.

Another beauty reason to cut back on high-GI carbohydrates is that they lead to weight gain, simply because they enter the body as sugar very quickly, raising your level of insulin, and any excess kilojoules that aren't required immediately are converted and stored as fat. Insulin is actually a fat storage hormone, and elevated levels of insulin put a 'fat lock' on our cellular fat-burning mechanism. Which explains why we can eat rice cakes, but not lose weight!

You'll find that along with stabilising your blood sugar levels, eating low-GI foods will help you fight fatigue, will increase your ability to concentrate and think clearly and will result in an improved sense of wellbeing.

Sea vegetables

The Japanese, renowned for their gorgeous skin, swear by sea vegetables, also known as seaweed. Sea vegetables are among the richest natural sources of minerals. It takes time to get used to using seaweeds, but they can make a tasty addition to your diet! Crush, chop, snip or crumble any mix of dried seaweeds you like into soups and sauces, casseroles, rice and salads. Roast them into anything you cook. If you add seaweed, you generally don't need salt. Sun-dried, they are convenient to buy, store and use as needed. Store them in a moisture-proof container and they will keep indefinitely.

Here's a quick profile of those most readily available.

Kelp (*Laminaria*) contains vitamins A, B, E, D and K and is a great source of vitamin C. It is also rich in minerals. Kelp works as a blood purifier, relieves arthritis stiffness and promotes adrenal, pituitary and thyroid health. Kelp's natural iodine can normalise thyroid-related disorders like obesity and lymph system congestion. Kelp is rich — a little goes a long way.

Kombu (*Laminaria japonica, setchelli*, horsetail kelp) has a long tradition as a Japanese delicacy with great nutritional healing value. It is a decongestant for excess mucous, and helps lower blood pressure. Kombu has abundant iodine, carotenes, B, C, D and E vitamins, minerals such as calcium, magnesium, potassium, silica, iron and zinc, and the powerful skin healing nutrient germanium. Kombu is a meaty, high-protein seaweed. Add a strip of kombu when cooking beans and legumes to reduce intestinal gas.

Hijiki (*Cystophyllum fusiforme*) is a mineral-rich, high-fibre seaweed that is 20 per cent protein, with vitamin A, carotenes and cal-cium. Hijiki has the most calcium of any sea green — 1400 milligrams per 100 grams of dry weight compared with 80 milligrams of calcium found in 100 grams of low-fat cottage cheese!

Nori (*Porphyra*, laver) is a red sea plant with a sweet, meaty taste when dried. It contains nearly 50 per cent balanced, assimilable protein, higher than any other sea plant. Nori's fibre makes it a perfect sushi wrapper. Nori is rich in all the carotenes, calcium, iodine, iron and phosphorus.

Arame (*Eisenia bycyclis*) is one of the ocean's richest sources of iodine. Herbalists use arame to help reduce breast and uterine fibroids. Through its fat-soluble vitamin and phytoestrogen action, it helps to normalise menopausal symptoms. Arame is believed to promote soft, wrinkle-free skin and enhances the shine, and prevents the loss of your hair.

Wakame (*Alaria, Undaria*) is a high-protein, high-calcium seaweed, with carotenes, iron and vitamin C. Widely used in the Orient for hair growth and lustre, and for skin tone.

Irish Moss (*Chondrus crispus*, carrageen) is full of electrolyte minerals — calcium, magnesium, sodium and potassium. Its compounds help to detoxify the body, boost metabolism and strengthen hair, skin and nails. It's traditionally used to improve a low sex drive.

 TIP

For a real beauty boost, drink one litre of water as soon as you wake. Elle McPherson and many other supermodels swear by it. Squeeze in some lemon for added zip. Keep a litre-size bottle close at hand, so you know how much you're actually drinking. Add a splash of your favourite juice, such as cranberry or apple, to it — this makes it all the more palatable and that way you'll drink more with less effort too!

Fantastic fluids

Last but certainly not least, water, and plenty of it, is an absolute must for gorgeous skin. Drinking at least eight glasses of pure water every day will leave your skin looking smoother, more hydrated and, as a result, visibly younger. Water is essential to maintain your skin's elasticity and suppleness, and it ensures proper hydration of the body, helping to reduce skin dryness. It's vital for diluting and expelling toxins, as well as helping to prevent blemishes. And don't think coffee or caffeinated soft drinks count; caffeine is dehydrating.

You can drink spring, sparkling, natural mineral or purified water. But avoid tap water; it contains a whole stack of heavy metals, fluoride, micro-organisms, and oxidising chlorine. Chlorine destroys your premier rejuvenating antioxidant vitamin E, which is crucial for gorgeous skin. Chlorine also has xenohormonic properties — meaning it can mimic hormones in your body.

So far you've taken in a lot of information — and your 30-day Gorgeous Skin program hasn't even begun! But it takes time to adjust to a new diet and eating habits, and this will be much more fun now that you're armed with a little background knowledge. It does take self-discipline to make healthy choices, but the rewards for your skin, in both the short and the long term, are enormous. It will get easier as you go along.

Cut kilojoules and take off years

Kilojoule restriction (or calorie restriction (CR) as it's also called) — obtaining optimal nutrition from the fewest kilojoules — has been studied for about seventy years in laboratory animals, primates and humans. The research has consistently reached the same conclusion: it extends life and reduces disease!

So what is kilojoule restriction? It's a lifestyle rather than a diet and requires that you eat about 10 to 15 per cent fewer kilojoules than it takes to maintain your weight according to standard BMI tables. The goal is to achieve a longer and healthier life by eating fewer kilojoules while maintaining and often improving nutrition. This means cutting out empty-joule foods and foods that are relatively high in joules but low in nutrients, such as simple sugars and flours, and replacing them firstly with lots of low-joule, high-nutrient foods like green leafy vegetables and high-fibre vegetables; secondly, with fruit; and thirdly with small amounts of fish, lean meat or other protein, such as nuts, beans, soy and eggwhite.

All kilojoule-restricted animals have certain things in common: they have lower levels of insulin, lower body temperatures and higher levels of DHEA (DHEA — dehydroepiandrosterone — is a natural hormone produced in our body by the adrenal glands; it's often referred to as the 'mother of the hormones' because it's further converted to generate a number of essential hormones). Interestingly, the one thing that the oldest living humans have in common is that they, too, have lower blood sugar levels and less insulin. Remember, insulin is a major accelerator of the ageing process.

Along with all the other potential health and longevity benefits, new research on kilojoule restriction offers promising results for skin ageing too! A study published in the January 2005 *American Medical Association Journal Archives of Facial Plastic Surgery* showed that restricting the dietary kilojoules of laboratory rats helped delay or prevent some of the non-environmentally induced changes that occur in ageing skin![29] The joule-restricted rats also produced more collagen and elastin fibres, fibroblasts (the mother cells of collagen and elastin) and capillaries than rats that were allowed to eat unlimited amounts of food. Although skin ageing in rats and humans isn't exactly identical, the possibility of cutting kilojoules to influence the rate of ageing is certainly worthy of attention.

According to the research so far, by maximising the 'nutrient density' of food intake, kilojoule restrictors not only enjoy a healthier life but anticipate a longer one as well. It's certainly food for thought!

3

Superfoods

How to Turbo-charge Your Beauty

In the last chapter we've discussed how eating for beauty will give your skin the nutrients it needs to repair itself and will enhance the blood supply to the dermis — your skin's deepest layer, keeping it supple and radiant. We've also seen how it will help to speed up the repair and regeneration of cells, to transport nutrients and to eliminate waste and toxins efficiently.

Now that we've looked at the nuts and bolts of nutrition for your skin, let's see which specific foods will do you the ultimate good and how much of each will benefit you most.

The 'superfoods' for gorgeous skin are natural, whole foods and extracts that supply an abundance of nourishing natural vitamins, minerals, healthy fats, amino acids, plant enzymes, antioxidants and phytonutrients. Each of the superfoods discussed in this chapter packs a powerful anti-ageing punch, and boasts more wrinkle-fighting promise than others. These nutrient superstars will enhance your skin's appearance and condition in a number of ways. They will:

- neutralise the effects of free radicals that can attack your skin's collagen and elastin
- enhance repair and regeneration of your skin cells
- subdue inflammation
- bump up cellular defence
- boost collagen production
- stimulate circulation to your skin's surface.

By making these superfoods part of your daily diet, you'll be eating your way towards your best skin yet. So start eating pretty!

The best beauty foods of all
Berries — your best wrinkle fighters

Berries are loaded with vitamins, minerals and powerful phytonutrient antioxidants that can help slow down the ageing process. Berries are a fantastic source of polyphenols, a class of phytonutrient antioxidants currently being studied for their anti-ageing power. Blueberries are the ultimate 'youth berries' as they pack three times the antioxidant punch of an orange. In fact, just one serving of blueberries provides as many antioxidants as five servings of carrots, apples, broccoli or squash! And just two-thirds of a cup of blueberries gives you the same antioxidant protection as 1733 IU of vitamin E and more protection than 1200 milligrams of vitamin C! A hefty handful of strawberries has all the antioxidant vitamin C your body requires each day to help reconstruct your collagen, the scaffolding that keeps your skin firm. One cup of strawberries provides over 125 per cent of the recommended dietary intake (RDI) of vitamin C, all for a skinny 190 kilojoules.

Blueberries and blackberries are rich in proanthocyanidins, which are potent, free-radical scavengers that guard your collagen and boost its repair. Proanthocyanidins also maintain the strength of your capillary walls (your capillaries are microscopic blood vessels that allow oxygen, hormones and nutrients to pass from your bloodstream to individual cells, including your skin cells) and, in doing so, protect capillaries at your skin's surface.

Beauty dosage: Eat one or more half-cup servings daily — about thirty berries — for gorgeous skin. Berries are typically treated with lots of pesticides, so where possible, go organic.

Beauty serving suggestions: Throw a handful of fresh or frozen blueberries or strawberries into your morning smoothie. Start the day with mixed berries, natural yoghurt and a few chopped almonds.

Rockmelon — foils flakiness

This colourful melon (one variety of which is the cantaloupe) is full of carotene compounds that help reduce the deep-down collagen damage that promotes wrinkles. A great source of beta-carotene (which is converted to vitamin A), rockmelon helps prevent keratonic plugs, the rough patches that sometimes develop on the backs of the arms. Rockmelon is also a dieter's delight! It's extremely low in kilojoules, has almost zero fat and its flavour is fantastic. A quarter of a medium rockmelon has about 210 kilojoules and provides 80 per cent of the RDI for both vitamins A and C. Rockmelon is higher in both these vitamins than honeydew or other winter melons.

Beauty dosage: Eat a few slices of rockmelon at least three times a week.

Beauty serving suggestions: Start your day with a few slices of rockmelon and slow-cooked oatmeal. Have a few slices with mixed berries for dessert.

Citrus fruits — collagen boosters

The collagen fibres that give your skin its elasticity can be improved by regular consumption of bioflavonoids and vitamin C, found in sizeable servings of citrus fruits like grapefruit and oranges and in kiwifruit, onions and capsicums. Vitamin C and bioflavonoids fend off free radicals and help guard your collagen. Citrus fruits also contain another powerful group of phytonutrients called the flavones, which bolster your antioxidant defence.

Beauty dosage: Eat one piece of citrus fruit daily.

Beauty serving suggestions: Start the day with a whole grapefruit cut in half. Don't forget to eat the inner white membranes, as they're brimming with bioflavonoids. Pink grapefruits make a tasty change and they're packed with the powerful phytonutrient lycopene (also found in tomatoes, guavas and watermelon). Instead of reaching for a chocolate bar or sweet treat, eat an orange and a handful of raw, unsalted almonds.

Prunes and plums – complexion perfection

Prunes, a great source of fibre, have long been recognised as a nutrient-rich fruit with multiple health benefits. According to a recent study from Tufts University in Boston, prunes may also help slow the ageing process. The study ranked the antioxidant value of commonly eaten fruits and vegetables using an analysis called Oxygen Radical Absorbance Capacity (ORAC) (see page 63). Prunes top the list, with more than twice the level of antioxidants than other high-scoring fruits such as blueberries and raisins. In fact, prunes are so powerful that they boost blood antioxidant levels by 25 per cent.

The ORAC values of dark-coloured fruits and vegetables are higher than lighter coloured ones; the darker and more intense the colour, the more antioxidant protection that's offered. The deep pigments of prunes and plums (along with dark grapes) are brimming with age-defying antioxidants and the phytonutrients carotenoids and polyphenols, both potent antioxidants.

Beauty dosage: Two prunes or plums (when in season) daily. Rinse but don't peel plums, as the skin is high in phytonutrients.

ORAC units for top-scoring antioxidant fruits & vegetables

FRUITS	UNITS PER 100G	VEGETABLES	UNITS PER 100G
Prunes	5570	Kale	1770
Raisins	2830	Spinach	1260
Blueberries	2400	Brussels sprouts	980
Blackberries	2036	Alfalfa sprouts	930
Strawberries	1540	Broccoli florets	890
Raspberries	1220	Beetroot	840
Plums	949	Red capsicum	710
Oranges	750	Onions	450
Red grapes	739	Corn	400
Cherries	670	Eggplant	390
Kiwi fruit	602		
Grapefruit, pink	483		

Source: UC Berkeley Wellness Letter, November 1999 [30]

For anti-ageing protection it's recommended that we consume between 3000 and 5000 ORAC units a day. This isn't as much as it sounds — half a cup of blueberries, for instance contains 2400 units. Try to eat both fruits and vegetables.

Beauty serving suggestions: Add prunes to mixed berries, slivered almonds and natural yoghurt for a great start to the day. Trade your morning or afternoon tea biscuits for succulent, ripe plums in season.

Broccoli — helps keep skin elastic

This sensational skin food packs the highest levels of antioxidant vitamins A and C in any food, as well as skin-cancer fighting chemicals. Vitamin C helps keep your skin elastic and prevents bruising.

Microwaving kills antioxidants

A study published in 2003 in the *Journal of the Science of Food and Agriculture* found that microwaved vegetables lose huge amounts of antioxidants.[31] Microwaved broccoli loses between 74 per cent and 97 per cent of its key antioxidant compounds. By stark contrast, steamed broccoli loses up to 11 per cent of the same antioxidants when these leach into the cooking water during heating.

Microwaves not only cause great losses in antioxidants, but they may pose other health threats too as they may bring about unnatural changes in food. Traditional methods of cooking involve radiant heat making its way into the food and cooking it from the outside in. Microwave ovens, on the other hand, generate an alternate current, causing food molecules to gyrate quite unnaturally billions of times each second. All this movement creates frictional heat, effectively cooking the food from the inside out.

Research published in *The Lancet* found that microwaving milk led to structural changes in the proteins that might well pose hazards for the body.[32] Some scientists have suggested that one particular protein formed in this way (D-proline) is toxic to the nervous system, kidneys and liver. In 1989, Swiss research also revealed that consuming food thawed and/or cooked in a microwave oven could cause undesirable changes in blood chemistry, such as a reduction in levels of haemoglobin (which can predispose to anaemia), and an increase in the number of immune cells in the bloodstream (generally taken to be a sign of stress, infection or inflammation).[33] At the moment, even though there is no irrefutable proof that microwaved food is hazardous to your health, I'd recommend using other methods of cooking.

Vitamin A aids in healing acne from the inside out by boosting resistance to infections. Broccoli also contains isothiocyanates, another powerful group of phytonutrients, which enhance the action of your detoxifying enzymes. One large cooked stalk has one and a half times your daily need for vitamin C, half your RDI for vitamin A, a small shot of B vitamins, and iron, calcium and fibre — all for just 110 kilojoules.

Beauty dosage: A few florets or a large stalk of broccoli every other day. (Opt for organic broccoli where possible as broccoli florets are great collectors of pesticides and other chemicals.)

Beauty serving suggestions: Lightly steam (in a minimum of water) or eat raw to get the most benefits. Include in salads, in stir-fries or with other vegetables.

Carrots — skin saver extraordinaire

Crunch all you want — carrots are bursting with beta-carotene which your body turns into skin-smoothing vitamin A, a key to keeping dry, flaky skin at bay. You'll also find beta-carotene in other orange fruits and vegetables, such as apricots and sweet potatoes.

According to Ronald R. Watson, PhD, professor of public health research at Arizona Health Sciences Centre in Tucson, 'beta-carotene accumulates in the skin, providing 24-hour protection against sun damage'.[34] Carrots are filled with other carotenoids (such as alpha-carotene) that also reduce UV damage to skin tissue, protect against free radical damage and enhance your skin's integrity through conversion to vitamin A. One carrot has double your RDI for vitamin A, plus it's fibre-rich and virtually fat-free.

Beauty dosage: One carrot per day (juiced, raw, grated or cooked).

Beauty serving suggestions: Finely grate raw carrots over leafy greens for a beta-carotene boost. Try carrot juice (mixed with apple and ginger for added zing) a few times a week for a gorgeous glow. Both juicing and grating break down the hard cell walls of the carrots, freeing the beta-carotene and making this nutrient easier to absorb.

 TIP

Beta-carotene is fat-soluble. To enhance its absorption, drizzle a little nut, olive or seed oil over raw or lightly steamed carrots and other vegetables containing beta-carotene.

Dark green leafy vegetables — the all-star antioxidants

Kale (closely followed by spinach) has one of the highest phyto-nutrient concentrations of all vegetables. These richly coloured leafy greens are packed with phytonutrient antioxidants like lutein and zeaxanthin. Other dark, leafy greens include rocket, beet greens, chard, collard greens, mustard greens, cos lettuce, turnip greens and watercress. Each contains a sizeable serving of zinc. In one Swedish study, acne-prone patients who added a zinc supplement to their diets saw 85 per cent of pimples clear up after three months.[35] Zinc is a must for gorgeous skin, as it helps break down damaged collagen, allowing new collagen to form. Zinc is also vital for normal cell growth. Dark-green leafy vegetables are a great source of iron too; iron has the all-important task of transporting oxygen to your skin. Dark circles under the eyes can be a sign of iron deficiency. They can also be caused by allergies — and, of course, insufficient sleep.

Beauty dosage: Eat two or more half-cup servings of spinach, kale or other dark, leafy greens per day.

Beauty serving suggestions: Toss baby spinach, rocket, collard greens or other dark leafy greens into a salad. Steam kale or spinach and drizzle with olive oil. Add kale or spinach or other greens to your juice to give it an added beauty boost. Cook with a little oil to up your lutein absorption.

 TIP

Raw garlic can sometimes leave you reaching for a serious shot of breath freshener. Munch on parsley, another great skin food, as it's loaded with chlorophyll, a natural breath freshener. Alternatively, take odourless garlic supplements to get the full benefit.

Garlic — glow-getter

Make garlic a daily ritual; it contains sulphur compounds that are a must for gorgeous skin and also potent phytonutrients that scavenge free radicals. Garlic boosts your immune system and is a powerful antibiotic, plus it's a great detoxifier. When cut, grated, pressed, crushed or chewed, fresh garlic releases enzymes that in turn trigger a cascade of beneficial chemical reactions inside your body. All this results in the formation of more than 200 phytonutrient compounds, each of which has impressive powers.

Beauty dosage: Go for one clove a day.

Beauty serving suggestions: Eat garlic raw, steamed or roasted. Use it to give flavour to almost any dish, including fish, vegetables and beans. Chop it up or mince it, then toss into salads and stir-fries. To give your dressings zest, add a clove of crushed garlic.

Parsley — an underrated skin food

Parsley is a culinary multi-vitamin. Each little sprig contains loads of nutrients, such as beta-carotene, B1, chlorophyll, calcium, and more vitamin C than citrus fruit. It contains just about all other known nutrients, including the hard-to-get B vitamin folic acid, which is important for pregnant women and those on the contraceptive pill, whose needs are almost doubled. Folic acid helps keep your skin tone vibrant, as it plays a key role in the formation and maturation of red blood cells. In fact, a pale, sallow complexion is one sign of folic acid deficiency anaemia. Half a cup of parsley delivers your entire daily need for folic acid, and offers a sizeable serving of vitamin C. It's also an excellent source of iron. Gram for gram, parsley has twenty-five times more iron than liver!

Beauty dosage: Think big! A whole bunch or half a bunch three times a week.

Beauty serving suggestions: Toss a whole chopped parsley bunch into a mixed green salad or sprinkle over vegies or fish. Stir parsley into soups and sauces just before serving. Add a bunch to your carrot 'skin-saver' juice.

Tomatoes – skin shaders

These sun-ripened fruits provide powerful UV protection for your skin. Tomatoes contain the potent free-radical scavenging phytonutrient lycopene (lycopene is the pigment that makes tomatoes and watermelon red, and pink grapefruit pink). Recent studies have revealed that lycopene may pack twice the punch of the well-known antioxidant beta-carotene. Tomatoes are also bursting with vitamin C. Many of the phytonutrient antioxidants (especially beta-carotene, lycopene and lutein) are credited with protecting your skin against sun damage and skin cancer.

When choosing your tomatoes, be sure to pick those with the most brilliant shades of red, as these indicate the highest amounts of beta-carotene and lycopene.

Beauty dosage: One whole tomato a day.

TIP

A big bonus is that, unlike many other phytonutrients, lycopene is relatively heat stable, so you can enjoy tomato sauce and tomato paste in casseroles soups and stews. You can also sauté tomatoes in olive oil to enhance your uptake of lycopene, which is a fat-soluble phytonutrient.

Beauty serving suggestions: Drizzle a small amount of olive oil over tomatoes. Eat them as a fruit. Bake them with basil. Cut them into salads or turn them into salsa. Use stewed tomatoes as a side dish or as a sauce for zucchini. Add tomato paste or tomato purée to soups, stocks or stews as an enricher.

Herbs – the antioxidant accessories

Fresh herbs such as rosemary, sage, oregano and thyme can be used to add colour and flavour to your cooking. And, for a built-in beauty bonus, they are all potent antioxidants.

Beauty serving suggestions: Chop fresh herbs and toss into salads or over fish or vegetables. Drizzle with olive oil. Ginger, a powerful antioxidant, can also add zest to food.

The power of raw: anti-ageing enzymes

Go raw for gorgeous skin. Raw food is rich in natural enzymes that contribute to fantastic health and great skin in so many ways. Enzymes are like your body's labour force: you need them for just about every process. They are vital sparks that initiate each chemical reaction. In fact, without enzymes, your vitamins, minerals and hormones would not be able to do their work and you wouldn't be able to digest your food. Balanced hormones, along with great digestion, absorption and assimilation of nutrients are critical for gorgeous skin.

It is believed that our bodies have a finite supply of enzymes and that this limited supply must last us a lifetime. It's just as though you inherited a certain amount of money. If you made all withdrawals and no deposits you would eventually run out of your inheritance.

It's estimated that our bodies naturally generate about 25 per cent of the enzymes we need for proper digestion, but the rest are expected to come from our diet. The problem is that the typical Western diet doesn't contain enough raw food to provide the missing 75 per cent or so of enzymes. When you cook food over 118 degrees Celsius, most of the beneficial enzymes are destroyed. Some enzymes are even destroyed by as little as 105 degrees, which means they may not survive even light steaming. When these natural enzymes are destroyed, your body has to generate the whole 100 per cent of enzymes necessary to digest the cooked food, so it needs to 'withdraw' enzymes from the 'bank'.

Some experts believe that it's this strain on our enzyme bank, caused by a diet of mostly cooked food, that is a paramount cause of premature ageing (and many degenerative diseases). Cells stop dividing, our immune system fails to handle challenges it once managed easily and our digestion becomes compromised. This is why an 85-year-old woman has 1/30 the enzyme activity level of an 18-year-old woman.

Professor Hans Eppinger, at the University of Vienna in Austria, discovered that a diet high in raw food significantly improves intra-cellular exchange, microcirculation and waste elimination. This means nutrients carried through the bloodstream via the capillaries make their way to your skin cells more efficiently, wastes are exchanged and your circulation is boosted. Natural enzymes also encourage the full assimilation of some of your important beauty vitamins and minerals. So have a fresh, raw salad instead of cooked vegetables, and raw fruit instead of dried.

 TIP

Eat raw food at least once a day. Start your meal with a little raw food to get your enzymes going and your digestive system primed.

Olive oil — the Greek wrinkle cure!

Dose up on olive oil for smooth, supple skin. Rich in mono-unsaturated fats and the phytonutrient antioxidant polyphenols, olive oil is a vital part of your daily anti-ageing arsenal. A study published in 2001 in the *Journal of the American College of Nutrition* examined the effects of diet on wrinkles.[36] Researchers compared the diets and skin of people living in sun-exposed areas and found that those with high intakes of olive oil, vegetables and legumes had the least wrinkling.

TIP

Always make sure you buy cold-pressed extra-virgin or virgin olive oil. This is unrefined and made with the highest quality olives, without using heat. These days, delicious organic olive oils from Italy, Spain, Greece, Australia and California are easy to find. Olive oil is also your best bet for cooking; the polyphenols protect against oxidation so it's relatively heat stable.

Beauty dosage: One to two tablespoons of olive oil daily.

Beauty serving suggestions: Add to salads. Drizzle over vegetables with fresh herbs and crushed pumpkin seeds. Use for sautéing and cooking.

Flaxseed oil and flax seeds — full of fantastic fatty acids

Flaxseed oil and flax seeds are an excellent source of the skin-softening Omega-3 (and to a lesser extent the Omega-6 fatty acids), as well as carotene and vitamin E, nutrients that feed healthy skin. Your cell membranes are mainly composed of essential fats, and the quality of the fats you eat shows directly on your skin's surface. Flaxseed oil keeps the skin soft and supple. Flax seeds (but not the oil) contain a great deal of fibre and, as a bonus, are the most abundant source of protective phytonutrient compounds called lignans. Lignans also act as phytoestrogens, which help to balance your body's hormones and keep your skin soft and youthful.

Freshly pressed flaxseed oil is sweet and nutty. But it's unstable: it oxidises (goes rancid and creates free radicals) rapidly when exposed to oxygen. By the time it gets to your table, it can have the undertone of oil paint! Always look for refrigerated flaxseed oil in small opaque bottles in your health-food store, always use it within six weeks of opening (and before the use-by date) and never heat it.

 TIP

You need to grind flax seeds to access their beneficial EFAs; if you eat them whole, they'll pass straight through you. Buy flax seeds in bulk and grind them to a coarse meal (but only as you use them) in a coffee grinder.

Beauty dosage: Two tablespoons of freshly ground flax seeds or one tablespoon of cold-pressed organic flaxseed oil daily.

Beauty serving suggestions: Sprinkle freshly ground flaxseeds over fresh fruit, vegetables or natural yoghurt. You can add a tablespoon of flaxseed oil or ground flax seeds to your morning smoothie.

Salmon – face-friendly fatty acids

This fish (especially caught in the wild) is teeming with face-friendly Omega-3 fatty acids, which do everything from attack dry areas to help deflate inflamed pimples. The essential fatty acids in wild salmon battle collagen-damaging free radicals and help smooth out fine lines. Omega-3s also help make eicosainoids, hormone-like substances that encourage our bodies to produce the human growth hormone (HGH). HGH is an anti-ageing hormone extraordinaire, as it boosts new cell growth.

HGH stimulates the growth of our tissues, our skin included, and it's one of the most important hormones for keeping us young. HGH is released by our pituitary gland and is converted in our liver to another anti-ageing hormone called insulin growth factor (IGF-1). Our body's production of HGH drops off steadily from our late twenties; by our sixties we have 50 per cent or less HGH in our bodies to promote healthy new cells.

Beauty dosage: An ideal amount of dietary Omega-3 fatty acids is about 7 grams per week, which you can obtain from two to three servings of fish. Eat cold-water, deep-sea fish such as mackerel, salmon, tuna and trout at least three times a week for smooth, supple skin. Where possible go for wild salmon in preference to farmed. If you don't enjoy seafood, or are a vegetarian, add one of the following for the same amount of Omega-3 fats as a 150g salmon fillet:

- 2 tablespoons walnut oil (cold pressed)
- 2 tablespoons soybean oil (cold-pressed, organic)
- 1 tablespoon canola oil (cold-pressed, organic)
- 3 tablespoons flaxseeds (ground)
- 4 tablespoons walnuts
- 1 cup soybeans (uncooked)
- 2000mg of a fish-oil (EPA/DHA) supplement.

Nuts — moisturise your skin from within

A primo source of monounsaturated fats, nuts moisturise your skin from the inside. The best nuts for your skin are almonds, walnuts and soy nuts. (Sunflower and pumpkin seeds are similarly beneficial.) Almonds contain great fats for your skin, protein, vitamin E, calcium and zinc — all important nutrients that keep your skin's outer layer (the epidermis) healthy. Walnuts are loaded with Omega-3 fatty acids for supple skin.

Beauty dosage: One to two tablespoons a few times a week.

Beauty serving suggestions: Toss a tablespoon of chopped walnuts into a salad or over vegetables. Add a few almonds to your morning smoothie. Grind up almonds or walnuts (in a coffee grinder) along with flax seeds for a fatty acid boost. Sprinkle steamed vegetables with fresh herbs and ground pumpkin seeds or sunflower seeds. For a satisfying snack, munch on dry-roasted soy nuts.

Avocados — beauty boosters

These great little packages of green contain something called glutathione — one of your master antioxidants and most powerful detoxifiers. Glutathione-rich avocados actually help cleanse your body of dangerous oxidised fats, and neutralise free radicals that can cause cell damage. Avocados are also loaded with phytonutrients — one of which is beta-sitosterol, which actually blocks the absorption of cholesterol into your bloodstream. Many people shun avocados for their high fat content, but they contain a healthy dose of mono-unsaturated fats — a major key to smooth, supple skin.

As an added skin bonus, avocados are also great nutrient boosters. They enhance your body's absorption of nutrients such as alpha-carotene, beta-carotene and lycopene found in other fruits and vegetables. So remember always to have good fat with your salads, and add avocado for an extra beauty boost.

Half a mature, medium-sized avocado contains about 630 kilojoules and fifteen grams of good monounsaturated fat. Avocados contain more potassium per gram than bananas, and they're a fair-to-good source of beta-carotene, vitamin E, vitamin C, folic acid and the important skin vitamin biotin.

Beauty dosage: Half an avocado a few times a week.

Biotin for beautiful skin

Biotin is an essential vitamin for fat synthesis — it's required for the function of the enzyme acetyl Co-A carboxylase, which puts together the building blocks for the production of fat in your body. A biotin deficiency can often show up as skin-related problems such as seborrheic dermatitis. Along with avocados, good sources of biotin include tomatoes, soybeans, whole grains and egg yolk.

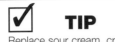

TIP

Replace sour cream, cream
cheese or butter with the
creamy goodness of avocados.

Beauty serving suggestions: Mash half an avocado on whole grain or dark rye bread. Dice an avocado into a leafy green salad and add walnuts.

Soy/tofu – skin saver

Whether in its original form (edamame) or transformed into tofu, the soy bean is a skin saver. It's a fantastic source of phytonutrients; in fact, there are about three hundred different phytonutrients in soy alone! The main ones in soy are a group called isoflavones, which include genistein and diadzin. These isoflavones are powerful anti-oxidants and have a protective phytoestrogenic action (see opposite).

Soy is also loaded with vitamin E, which boosts new cell growth and keeps skin moist. Like meat, soy is a complete protein, so it contains all your essential amino acids along with calcium and magnesium, but without the saturated fat. It also contains some skin-smoothing Omega-3 fatty acids.

Beauty dosage: Eat several servings of unprocessed and preferably fermented soy products a week to get their full benefits. One serving is a cup of soymilk, 85g of tofu, or 1/2 cup of tempeh or miso.

Beauty serving suggestions: Make organic soymilk or silken (soft) tofu the base of your morning smoothie. Throw a package of organic silken tofu into a blender with some fresh or frozen fruit for a super healthy breakfast. To pack a powerful punch of anti-ageing antioxidants, add a handful of blueberries, a few raw unsalted nuts such as walnuts or almonds, and a teaspoon of flaxseed oil. Tofu takes on the flavour of anything it's cooked with: add firm tofu to stir-fries, soups, curries and stews. It can also be grilled. Munch on edamame

What are phytoestrogens?

Phytoestrogens, or plant oestrogens, are very weak oestrogens that occur naturally in many plant foods. The chemical structure of these phytoestrogens is similar, but not identical, to the oestrogens produced by your body. Also the activity of phytoestrogens is generally much weaker than your own oestrogen (their estrogenic activity is between 1/500th and 1/1000th the activity of your own oestrogen).

These phytoestrogens can actually help protect you from potential damage by binding together with your body's oestrogen receptors. (Certain forms of oestrogens in your body can stimulate tumour formation and growth.) So phytoestrogens may prevent cancer-causing hormones from 'docking' in your cells where they do their dirty work by attaching themselves onto your receptors.

The Japanese, who consume an abundance of soy, have much lower rates of breast cancer than Australian women. This oestrogen-blocking action is thought to be one of the reasons for their lower incidence of breast cancer. Japanese men also have a much lower death rate due to prostate cancer, which may also be linked to their high soy intake.

(whole green soybeans boiled in their skins for ten minutes in salty water) or dry-roasted soy nuts.

Not a soy fan? Not to worry. There are plenty of other ways to add the phytoestrogen phytonutrients to your diet for their protective benefits.

Phytonutrient Class	Sources
Isoflavones	Soybeans, tempeh, tofu, soy milk, miso (soy sauce isn't a significant source of isoflavones)
Flavanols	Onions, lettuce, tomatoes, red wine, green tea
Flavones	Apples, green tea
Flavanones	Citrus peels
Lignans	Flax seed or flax flour, lentils; small amounts are also found in garlic, squash and asparagus

Oatmeal — ousts toxins

Go for slow-cooked oats, not the instant kind. You'll get a dose of fibre that, once converted, helps filter toxins and raises your clear-skin potential. Oats are rich in B vitamins, which aid new cell-growth. Oats are also a wonderful source of calcium, iron, magnesium, potassium, silicon, vitamin E, the B vitamins and protein.

You get two kinds of fibre from oats — insoluble and soluble. Insoluble fibre keeps you regular; soluble fibre helps stabilise your blood-sugar levels so that emotions also stay on an even keel. How does that help your skin? Constipation and mood swings can be a source of stress, and any stress-inducers can precipitate skin eruptions.

Beauty dosage: A few times a week.

Beauty serving suggestions: Choose slow-cooking oatmeal for breakfast. Add soymilk, crushed nuts and berries or a few slices of rockmelon.

Spirulina — skin treat

Spirulina is a fresh-water, blue–green algae that's an ideal skin and anti-ageing food: it has a concentrated nutrient value, is easily digested, loaded with antioxidants and a good source of usable protein, B vitamins (including B12), beta-carotene, essential fatty acids and chlorophyll — all required for radiant skin. In fact, spirulina is the richest food source of beta-carotene, with a full spectrum of ten mixed carotenoids that all work synergistically at different sites in your body to enhance your antioxidant protection. Spirulina also helps stabilise blood sugar levels, which decreases the need for those emergency chocolate bars and chips that so often trigger problem skin.

Beauty dosage: One teaspoon of powdered spirulina or six to twelve (organic) spirulina tablets daily. You can add powdered spirulina to juice, water or your smoothie. Because spirulina is a whole food, it can be taken alone or with meals.

Supporting stars

Here's an A to Z of other foods that are excellent for your skin. They should play a supporting role in any beauty regimen.

- apples
- apricots
- asparagus
- beans (black, kidney, lima)
- beetroot
- brown rice
- brussels sprouts
- cabbage
- capsicum (all kinds)
- cauliflower
- celery
- clams
- coconut oil
- cottage cheese
- cucumbers
- eggs
- endive
- honeydew melon
- kiwi fruit
- lentils
- macadamia nut oil
- mangos
- mushrooms
- natural yoghurt
- paw paw
- pears
- skinless chicken (free range)
- squash
- turkey breast
- zucchini

What you choose to eat on a daily basis has a cumulative effect. Making bad food choices can show up in days, months or sometimes even years as age spots, sagging or sallow skin, wrinkles, dryness, broken capillaries, poor skin tone and premature ageing. Eating a wide variety of the superfoods daily is a major key to achieving great skin. The micronutrients, antioxidants, phytonutrients and essential fats and protein found in these foods, feed your skin cells, help build your skin's internal scaffolding, accelerate the repair process and reduce the appearance of fine lines, wrinkles, uneven pigmentation, broken capillaries, dryness, under-eye circles and puffiness. By becoming a devotee of antioxidant, phytonutrient nutrient-rich foods, you'll be on your way to achieving your best ever skin, not only now, but in the future.

4

Nutritional Supplements

Maximising Skin Rejuvenation

Remember that your skin contains rich stores of antioxidants because it's your body's first line of defence against free radicals. It is also made up of rapidly dividing cells, making it especially sensitive to nutrient levels. These nutrients have a long way to get to the tiny capillaries that feed your skin, so skin cells need all the extra nutritional support they can get.

The second tier of the Gorgeous Skin program is the introduction of nutritional supplements. They're an absolute must during the 30-day program, as they'll really help maximise the effects of skin rejuvenation. Supplements can't replace a great diet, but they can certainly boost the effects of a healthy diet to promote beauty from the inside. Plus, they can help slow down the visible signs of ageing.

These days even if we do have a great diet, we still live in an imperfect world — we're bombarded by pollution, environmental chemicals and second-hand smoke, along with the stresses of modern-day life. And the food we eat just isn't what it used to be, even if you stick to a great wholefood, organic diet.

In this chapter, each of the key supplements we'll be looking at is specifically designed to combat free radicals, decrease inflammation and promote the development of healthy skin cells. A great complexion is the result of millions of cells working efficiently thanks to a continuing supply of micronutrients, essential fats, first-rate protein, phytonutrients and antioxidants. Without question, a nutrient-rich diet plus supplements are your best bets for achieving a youthful complexion for life.

But why is a good diet not enough? The answer is both an agricultural and an environmental one. For a start, our topsoil (the nutrient-rich ground cover) just doesn't contain the levels of nutrients it used to. Recent farming trends fertilise the soil with synthetic chemicals instead of manure and compost, and this depletes nutrients. Poor rotation of crops also leads to erosion and nutrient depletion. All this ultimately means that we end up with less nutrition in the food we eat.

Along with a depletion of vital antioxidants, trace minerals and phytonutrients, a lot of food today contains harmful levels of pesticides and other toxic chemicals. The vast majority of what we eat also tends to be overly processed, refined and stripped of its nutritional value. The fatty acid profile of fish and meat has altered dramatically over the last few decades too, favouring the Omega-6 fatty acids (which, in excess, promote inflammation) over the Omega-3s. So we just aren't getting the nutrients from our food like we did as recently as a few decades ago.

What does this all mean for your skin? Deficiencies of certain vitamins and minerals such as vitamins C and A, zinc, selenium and essential fatty acids are particularly detrimental to the skin and can result in skin disorders/diseases and accelerated ageing. This is because micronutrients are needed for just about every single process in your body, including the manufacture of anti-ageing hormones, optimal mitochondrial (your cell powerhouses) function, protection against free radical and DNA damage and the maintenance of cell function at peak levels. A deficiency of certain nutrients, including folic acid, B3, iron, zinc or vitamins B12, B6, C or E, appears to mimic radiation by causing breaks in your DNA strands. While severe vitamin and mineral deficiencies are rare in developed countries like Australia, mild deficiencies are surprisingly common. Added to that, as we age we absorb vitamins and minerals less efficiently, so extra protection is absolutely critical. In fact, these days most people need — and thrive on — added nutrients in the form of supplements.

Nutritionists aren't the only ones advocating supplements for gorgeous skin. Many dermatologists are now favouring oral dietary supplements along with topical treatments, and even companies like Olay are creating their own lines of internal skin supplements. Renowned Los Angeles dermatologist Dr Ronald Moy has pointed out that antioxidant supplements are more effective than topical treatments because, when taken internally, antioxidants go directly to the bloodstream rather than sitting on the skin's surface, far away from the dermis where wrinkles are formed. Also, he says, 'Topical antioxidants are notoriously unstable and when taking them internally you don't have to worry about a pill being broken down by light.'[37]

But can antioxidants (whether in supplement form or food form) really help create younger-looking skin? Definitely. As we've seen, free radical damage is one of the principal mechanisms of ageing. And remember, your skin contains a rich reserve of antioxidants, as it's the principal barrier between your body and pollution, cigarette smoke, ultraviolet rays, hazardous chemicals and other sources of free radicals. With age, however, the accumulation of environmental exposure to free radicals, plus the internal oxidation and breakdown of collagen, can cause skin to lose its tone and healthy glow. Internal antioxidants can help create younger-looking skin by reducing inflammation, fending off free radicals and inhibiting certain enzymes, such as hyaluronidase, which break down collagen.

A phytonutrient family called the proanthocyanidins, or OPCs, which are found in grapeseed extract, and Pycnogenol (pine bark extract) inhibit this enzyme hyaluronidase. Plus proanthocyanidins also strengthen capillaries — another great skin bonus. Some anti-oxidants such as N-acetyl-cysteine (NAC) even improve the rate at which collagen is created.

Some of the other antioxidants we'll be discussing include alpha-lipoic acid, vitamins A, C, and E, which together with selenium, zinc and l-cysteine help stop free radicals from oxidising the fatty layer of your skin cells, and in doing so help to protect your skin from damage and photo ageing. Just take vitamin C, for example: it protects against oxidative stress that occurs as a result of UV exposure. Vitamin C is also an essential co-factor in the creation of collagen, so even a slight deficiency of vitamin C can result in diminished collagen production.

Other antioxidants such as alpha-tocopherol (vitamin E) and the carotenoids such as beta-carotene, which are found in your skin cells, can also partially protect against photo ageing by shielding your skin cells from oxidative damage. Beta-carotene has been found to protect against UV-induced oxidative stress, and in doing so reduces skin damage.[38] So your daily carrot juice is also protecting your skin.

The skin supplements

On the Gorgeous Skin program you'll probably be taking more supplements than you're used to, and also more frequently. You also may be taking ones that you've never heard of before. To ensure that you maintain therapeutic levels in your blood, I recommend that you take the supplements more than once a day. One simple way to keep track is to use an inexpensive weekly pill or supplement sorter, available at your chemist. Make taking these supplements a habit — something you do automatically, without a second thought, like brushing your teeth. This may take some time and effort. But, if you understand the benefits and set your mind to it the rewards will be enormous.

Because beauty and health are inseparable, it's impossible to improve one without boosting the other. The best news is that by taking the supplements recommended here you'll be not only doing your skin a great favour but also improving your health and every organ system of your body.

A note on supplement quality

Do not assume that all vitamin supplements are the same quality; you generally get what you pay for. Avoid supplements that have 100 per cent of all the recommended dietary intakes (RDIs). They're useless. One little pill doesn't provide everything you need. Plus the RDIs are set so incredibly low, just barely enough to prevent you getting the disorder or deficiency sign associated with that vitamin. The RDI recommendations are also dated and don't guarantee good health. The most advanced full-spectrum multi-nutrient regimes contain therapeutically proven potencies of nutrients that far exceed the RDI. Another key factor is absorption. It's not what you take, but what you absorb, that counts. Food-like forms of supplements are absorbed best and this requires bulk.

To ensure that you buy quality, follow these three simple pointers.

- Avoid the cheapest vitamins, generic chemist or supermarket brands, and brands filled with di-calcium phosphate, cellulose and other fillers. A handful of studies show decreased absorption or benefit in certain synthetic vitamins, such as dl-alpha-tocopherol (the synthetic form of vitamin E). The d-alpha form has been shown to be more beneficial.
- Look for mixed carotenoids. Recent studies show that mixed carotenoids — not just beta-carotene by itself — work together

to protect the skin against the harmful effects of UV radiation and reduce DNA damage, one of the leading causes of many types of cancer.

- Look for mixed tocopherols rather than just alpha-tocopherol (vitamin E) and bioflavonoids such as quercetin rather than just vitamin C.

A note on safety

Quality vitamins and supplements should not cause health problems themselves. However, excessive use of individual supplements, particularly in synthetic form, may be unhealthy.

! You should always check with your health care provider or nutritionist before taking any new supplements, especially if you are taking prescription or over-the-counter medications.

———————■———————

While we need small quantities of every single essential nutrient for optimal health, your skin relies on some of these more than others for its wellbeing. In this next section, we'll look at the most important supplements for the skin and discuss their specific benefits. Although the list is far from exhaustive, these supplements are specifically targeted at disarming oxidation, preventing inflammation and feeding your skin with an array of valuable nutrients to build beautiful skin from within. The supplements listed in this section are some of the best researched and most highly regarded in the field of anti-ageing at the time of writing this book.

Antioxidants — the great anti-agers
Vitamin C — the wrinkle-fighting antioxidant

Description: Water-soluble vitamin and potent natural antioxidant. Humans are among only a handful of species on the planet that can't manufacture their own supplies of vitamin C, so we need to replenish our stores daily. Vitamin C is a water-soluble vitamin, so whatever supplies are not used immediately are quickly excreted in urine. In fact, the biochemical activity of vitamin C lasts only about six hours in your body, regardless of whether it is ingested as food or as supplements, so it's best to replenish this magnificent beauty promoter two to three times per day.

Skin beauty benefits: Vitamin C is one of the most important nutrients for protecting and preserving health and beauty. With special help from the bioflavonoids, vitamin C helps build collagen (it's an essential cofactor for the enzymes involved in making collagen), which gives your skin its youthful bounce. Vitamin C is also a spectacular antioxidant. Whenever vitamin C encounters a free radical, it sacrifices one of its own electrons in order to 'pacify' and neutralise the intruder, destroying itself in the process. This running battle between vitamin C and free radicals occurs hundreds of thousands of times per second. Vitamin C helps protect against the oxidative stress that occurs as a result of UV exposure, which can lead to photo ageing of the skin. Compared with healthy skin, photo-aged skin or naturally aged skin contains lower levels of vitamin C.

Vitamin C not only snags free radicals but recharges levels of vitamin E and glutathione peroxidase, also powerful antioxidants which can help your body fight the effects of pollution, smoking and radiation. Along with playing an important role in preventing ageing and skin wrinkling, easy bruising and broken veins under the skin, this anti-ageing vitamin also helps combat stress and varicose veins.

There is considerable evidence that supplemental vitamin C, plus a diet high in raw fruits and vegetables, helps save skin from premature ageing. But of all the dietary (from food and supplements) vitamin C absorbed by our bodies, only about 8 per cent is taken up by the skin. So you need ample amounts of vitamin C from both your diet and added supplements.

Deficiency symptoms: Easy bruising, bleeding gums when brushing or flossing, premature wrinkling, poor immunity to colds and flu.

Recommended daily beauty dosage: 500–2000mg (Take in divided doses throughout the day). Take vitamin C with bioflavonoids (bioflavonoids are often combined with vitamin C in supplements) as this increases the absorption of vitamin C by a whopping 35 per cent! As a water-soluble vitamin, vitamin C is extremely safe even at relatively high doses, as what doesn't get used generally gets excreted in the urine.

The recommended dietary intake (RDI) for vitamin C of 40mg is not even enough for normal nutritional needs, much less for viable protection from free-radical damage.

Smokers alert! If you are a smoker you're at particularly high risk of vitamin C deficiency. Each cigarette uses up about 25mg of vitamin C, a major reason why smokers lose collagen elasticity much faster than non-smokers!

Bioflavonoids – chief assistant to vitamin C

Description: Bioflavonoids are naturally occurring water-soluble plant substances that give fruits and vegetables their distinctive colours. Plus, they are powerful antioxidants in their own right. They are most commonly found with vitamin C in foods, and they enhance vitamin C's antioxidant capacity and are necessary for its absorption and utilisation. Bioflavonoids include the brightly coloured substances citrin, rutin, anthocyanidins, quercetin, proanthocyanidins, tangeritin, hesperidin, flavones and flavonals.

Skin beauty benefits: Bioflavonoids help keep your skin supple and elastic by assisting vitamin C in its role of making and preserving collagen. They are also an absolute must for healthy blood vessels! The bioflavonoids work by strengthening blood vessel walls and preventing and healing capillary breakage, which aids circulation and prevents haemorrhaging and ruptures in the skin. Bioflavonoids also help to tone small broken capillaries and varicose veins. They also regulate capillary permeability, and act as powerful antioxidants that protect cells and blood vessels from damage.

Deficiency symptoms: Bruising, spongy gums, fragile capillaries, varicose veins, wrinkles, sagging skin, premature ageing, poor immunity and slow healing.

Recommended daily beauty dosage: 600–3000mg of mixed bioflavonoids.

Vitamin E — youth and beauty preserver

Description: Vitamin E is a powerful fat-soluble antioxidant that protects cell membranes from oxidative damage. Technically, vitamin E is known as tocopherol but it actually exists in eight different forms. There are four different tocopherols and four tocotrienols. Tocopherols are the more familiar forms of vitamin E, but tocotrienols have additional functions and health benefits. Each form has its own biological activity. The tocopherols are differentiated by one of the first four letters of the Greek alphabet — alpha, beta, gamma and delta. Alpha-tocopherol is the most active or usable form of vitamin E for your body.

Skin beauty benefits: This spectacular antioxidant helps to counteract premature ageing by protecting your cellular membranes and other 'oily' structures from damage and genetic mutation. Vitamin E sits in the membrane and acts as a security guard ready to pounce on free radicals. As 'oily' molecules are especially susceptible to free radical damage, vitamin E is important in helping protect your skin from environmental damage and other assaults. When free radicals come along, they hitch up to vitamin E, damaging it instead of the rest of the cell membrane. In the process, vitamin E soaks up free radicals and the cell is protected from damage. Also, unless liberally supplied with vitamin E, these membranes can lose flexibility, harden and age. They then stop taking in nutrients and discharging wastes efficiently, which is bad news for skin.

Vitamin E also oxygenates tissues and increases your body's stores of vitamin A. It can prolong cell life, promote healing and reduce scarring. In addition vitamin E has been shown to improve a variety of skin conditions, including acne, eczema, and psoriasis. Plus, it's a valuable treatment for sunburn. Vitamin C and other antioxidants can regenerate vitamin E. But with a shortage of vitamin E, there's an increase in free radicals, cellular injuries and subsequent disorders to bodily tissues, including accelerated ageing of the skin. Vitamin E works best in combination with selenium and vitamin C.

Deficiency symptoms: Premature ageing, lacklustre skin, lethargy and muscle wasting.

Recommended daily beauty dosage: 400–800 International Units (IU) daily. Beware of dl-alpha-tocopherol — it's a synthetic form of vitamin E and not well recognised by your body. Look for mixed tocopherols and tocotrienols. Vitamin E is probably the most challenging vitamin to obtain through diet alone because even the richest beauty food sources fall short of the recommended dosage.

! Top up on vitamin E when your skin is exposed to sun.

! If you have high blood pressure or are taking blood thinners (such as the anticoagulant medication Warfarin), consult your doctor before taking vitamin E. Vitamin E is a mild anticoagulant (blood thinner) so you must inform and consult with your health care provider before any surgery.

Vitamin A – wrinkle fighter extraordinaire

Description: Vitamin A is a fat-soluble vitamin and antioxidant. Your body can store vitamin A, so you must be cautious of an excessive intake of the supplement. In extremely high doses it can lead to toxicity.

Skin beauty benefits: The number one wrinkle-fighter, vitamin A is critical for the normal growth, development and renewal of skin cells, keeps skin tissue healthy and is a powerful antioxidant. By nurturing the fat lying beneath the skin, vitamin A helps ensure that skin is taut, silky soft and youthful looking. Vitamin A also makes sure that the skin cells rising to the surface remain supple, so your skin feels soft and smooth. Vitamin A may help prevent sun damage.

Deficiency symptoms: It's time to top up on vitamin A if your skin is dry or rough, or it breaks out in spots. Other deficiency signs include dry, fragile skin prone to wrinkles, blackheads, white heads, splitting nails, bumpy and pimply skin.

! If you're deficient in vitamin A, no skin treatment will work properly!

Recommended daily beauty dosage: 10,000–25,000 International Units (IU) or up to 50,000 IUs under the supervision of a medical practitioner. If pregnant or trying to become pregnant, keep dosages below 10,000 IUs.

! Take a teaspoon of cold-pressed cod liver oil every day, especially during the winter months — it's also a wonderful source of vitamin D.

! It's important to top up on vitamin A when your skin is exposed to strong sun.

! **Vitamin A toxicity alert:** Excessive amounts of vitamin A (particularly synthetic vitamin A) can overload tissues and cause toxicity. A much safer way to keep an optimum level is to increase mixed carotenoids, including beta-carotene intake.

Beta-carotene — beauty booster and sun shader

Description: Beta-carotene, derived from the Latin name for carrot, belongs to the phytonutrient family known as carotenes or carotenoids. There are more than 600 carotenoids in nature, found mostly in orange and yellow fruits and vegetables and dark-green vegetables. Beta-carotene was the first carotenoid to be isolated and is the most widely studied. Once eaten, beta-carotene is converted to vitamin A (retinol) in the body when needed. It's a powerful antioxidant in its own right.

Skin beauty benefits: Beta-carotene helps your body generate new cells, including skin cells, and protects against cancer. It also helps prevent dry, rough skin and premature ageing. As an antioxidant its main role is to detoxify a highly energetic free radical called the Singlet oxygen free radical. The Singlet oxygen free radical is produced as a natural by-product of metabolism as well as from exposure to UV rays, and it's particularly reactive and highly destructive to cells. Sunlight-induced Singlet oxygen mutates the DNA in your skin fibroblasts, and this accelerates extrinsic ageing. Beta-carotene is one of your best defences against these nasty free radicals. Its potent antioxidant properties also neutralise the very destructive polyunsaturated-fat radical. Plus, it speeds healing and is great for acne.

Certain carotenoids can act like 'shades' for your skin. Beta-carotene helps protect your skin from the free radicals produced from UV exposure and allows longer exposure to the sun without damage. The January 2003 issue of the US *Journal of Nutrition* reported that supplemental beta-carotene (along with vitamin E) can reduce susceptibility to sunburn. Vitamin E works synergistically with the carotenoids, boosting their effect. Beta-carotene quenches free radicals, which can promote inflammation and skin cell damage characteristic of sunburn. This study found that either a natural beta-carotene or mixed-carotenoid supplement (typical of the mix of carotenoids found in fruits and vegetables) provides similar protection against sunburn.[39] Scientists believe that beta-carotene works by causing slight changes in skin pigmentation and preventing free-radical damage to the skin. If you want the additional protection, vitamin E and carotenoid supplements should be taken over a four- to six-week period before increased sun exposure, as it takes several weeks for these nutrients to build up in the skin.

Deficiency symptoms: Premature wrinkles, acne, pimples, blackheads, psoriasis, vision disorders, respiratory problems, dry, rough, itchy, scaly, cracked skin and slowed healing. An early sign of beta-carotene deficiency is chicken skin — small raised bumps on the back of the neck, upper arms, back and shoulders.

Recommended daily beauty dosage: 15–160mg.

! If you exceed the recommended dosage for a long period of time, your skin may turn an orangey colour due to the beta-carotene accumulation in the fat layer underneath the dermis. Cut back and this will disappear.

! It's best to take this supplement in the mixed carotenoid form. Studies conducted in the mid-1990s in Finland and the United States found that beta-carotene supplements increased lung cancer risk in smokers. This study, however, used synthetic beta-carotene.

Coenzyme Q10 (CoQ10) – powerful free radical quencher

Description: Technically known as ubiquinone, coenzyme Q10 (CoQ10) is a powerful antioxidant found naturally inside cells. It protects the body from free radical damage and aids in metabolic reactions. It plays an essential role in energy production, as well as acting as an antioxidant in cell membranes. These membranes function as the doors and walls of cells, letting nutrients in and waste products out.

CoQ10 accelerates the action of your cell's motor — the mitochondria — keeping cells running like well-tuned cars while protecting your motor from destructive free radicals. When the mitochondria runs down, the ageing process can run rampant. Your mitochondria contain the greatest amount of CoQ10. Unfortunately, CoQ10 can also auto-oxidise — that is, it can become a free radical itself under some circumstances — but vitamin E can prevent this. Studies suggest that these two substances work synergistically, as do many other antioxidants, such as vitamins C, E, A and alpha-lipoic acid.

Skin beauty benefits: Your skin contains high levels of CoQ10. It's necessary for production of adenosine triphosphate (ATP), the 'fuel' of all living cells. The increased energy production facilitated by CoQ10 will benefit your skin as well. With age your body produces less CoQ10, so there is less of its antioxidant power to go around. This is bad news for skin cells because, in theory, low levels of

CoQ10 can show up as skin ageing. CoQ10 is sometimes called a 'biomarker of ageing' because its level correlates so well with ageing and degenerative diseases. Excessive exposure to ultraviolet radiation can rapidly deplete levels of CoQ10 in the skin.

Deficiency symptoms: A deficiency of CoQ10 has been associated with a variety of heart problems including arrhythmias, angina and high blood pressure. Gingivitis (inflammation of the gums) and problems in regulating blood sugar have also been linked to a CoQ10 deficiency.

Recommended daily beauty dosage: 30–200mg (take it with food as it's fat soluble).

! CoQ10 may intensify the effects of blood thinners such as Coumadin (Warfarin), so consult your medical practitioner before taking it.

Alpha lipoic acid – universal and potent antioxidant

Description: Alpha-lipoic acid is one of the most powerful anti-ageing antioxidants and anti-inflammatories available. As with many key substances in the body, levels of lipoic acid decline with age. It's both water- and fat-soluble, which means it can work in each and every part of your skin cells — in the fatty cell membranes and in the aqueous interior of your cells. Plus, it's amazingly effective in combating many different forms of oxidative stress and cellular damage in all parts of your cells. It terminates a free radical known as the hydroxyl radical, which happens to be one of the most damaging to the body. It also helps regenerate other antioxidants after they are 'used up' fighting free radicals.

According to one of the world's leading authorities on antioxidants, Dr Lester Packer of the University of California in Berkeley, 'lipoic acid is the most versatile and powerful antioxidant in the entire antioxidant defence network'.[40] Lipoic acid has an unusual relationship with four other important antioxidants: glutathione, coenzyme Q10, vitamin C and vitamin E. Dr Packer's extensive research has shown that together these five compounds form a unique 'antioxidant network': they interact with each other in such a way as to regenerate their antioxidant capacities after they have successfully neutralised free radicals. In other words, they can be used over and over again as antioxidants. Great news for your skin — as without this regenerative process, these molecules (like most other antioxidants) would be lost to metabolic processes once they have reacted with free radicals. Because lipoic acid is the linchpin in this process, it's the only one that can recycle the other four (and the only one that can do this by itself).

Skin beauty benefits: Alpha-lipoic acid preserves and boosts the level of antioxidants in the skin, shoring up defences against ageing. Most of the skin benefits are from its free radical fending action, as well as being strongly anti-inflammatory. Another great skin bonus is that lipoic acid improves insulin resistance and speeds the removal of glucose from your bloodstream. Plus, it has been shown to help neutralise and remove a variety of toxic metals from the body. It is also an inhibitor of glycation and cross-linking. (Remember glycation and cross-linking are key age accelerators.)

Recommended daily beauty dosage: 50–100mg twice a day. There is no recommended dietary intake (RDI) established for lipoic acid.

Acetyl L-Carnitine/L-Carnitine

Description: Acetyl L-Carnitine (ALC) is a naturally occurring amino acid related to L-Carnitine. You may have heard of this supplement for the treatment of Alzheimer's and Parkinson's disease. It protects and increases receptors (particularly for memory) in the brain that normally decline with age. It also increases energy levels in the body and enhances fatty acid transport.

Skin beauty benefits: Acetyl L-Carnitine has a whole stack of great skin benefits, too. It has been shown to counteract glycation, promote melatonin production, restore cortisol receptors, and boost levels of the key antioxidants glutathione and CoQ10. It also helps to dissolve lipofuscin (sometimes called the 'ageing pigment'). This brownish pigment increases with age and is left over from the breakdown and absorption of damaged blood cells.

Daily beauty dosage: 500–1000mg daily on an empty stomach.

! Best taken with alpha-lipoic acid, CoQ10 and other antioxidants.

! It works best when carbohydrates are minimised.

Carnosine – prevents cross-linking

Description: The new superstar in the fight against ageing, carnosine (not to be confused with 'carnitine') is a combination of two amino acids (building blocks of proteins): alanine and histidine. Carnosine was discovered more than a hundred years ago and it has been used in Russia for many years, but its specific anti-ageing properties have only recently come to light in the West.

Skin beauty benefits: It's a powerful water-soluble antioxidant, which has been shown to quench the most destructive of free radicals: the hydroxyl radical, along with superoxide, Singlet oxygen and the peroxyl radical. Most importantly it has a remarkable ability to help prevent cross-linking and glycation, both of which ultimately lead to a loss of elasticity as well as wrinkles and other signs of premature ageing.

! Glycated proteins produce fifty times more free radicals than non-glycated proteins and carnosine may be the most effective anti-glycating agent known.

Recommended daily beauty dosage: 500–1500mg. Unfortunately carnosine isn't available in Australia at the moment, but if you're keen to take it you can easily order it online from the United States. Suppliers are listed under Resources, page 306.

Essential fatty acids – beautifying fats

Description: Remember that the reason these fats are called 'essential' is that your body can't manufacture them; you must obtain them from the foods you eat or through supplements. EFAs fall into two categories, Omega-3 and Omega-6.

Skin beauty benefits: If you want to stop fine lines from appearing and to maintain moist, radiant skin, then essential fatty acids are the key. The beneficial effects of EFAs for improving skin are staggering. They have a powerful effect on hormones, improving blood flow, and are strongly anti-inflammatory. They help lubricate the fatty layer just beneath your skin. EFAs are also vital for wound healing, psoriasis and balancing sebum production (EFAs will improve your skin, whether it's oily or dry). When you supplement with the Omega-3s you'll definitely see a change in the texture of your skin, and you'll probably also notice a softening of the lines on your face.

Your skin requires a constant supply of EFAs, but it particularly needs EFAs when stressed by the damage that occurs with sunburn. Experiments have shown that UV rays cause a significant release of fatty acids from the cell membranes. The cells use these fatty acids to regulate the inflammation, swelling and pain. Gamma linolenic acid (GLA), from borage, evening primrose and black currant oils, has been found to reduce redness, swelling and pain from UV damage. Also as we age, GLA production decreases, and that's one reason we become more susceptible to wrinkles. Babies have higher levels of GLA, which is one of the reasons they have such plump, moist skin. A number of other factors diminish the amount of GLA in your body, including; hydrogenated fats, fried foods, sugar, a sluggish thyroid and low levels of magnesium, zinc and vitamins C, B3 and B6.

Deficiency symptoms: Dry, scaly skin, eczema, inflammatory skin conditions, slow healing. Also hair loss or thinning, dandruff, splitting nails and dull hair.

Recommended daily beauty dosage: 1–2 tablespoons of flaxseed oil, 500mg of GLA, 1000–3000mg of EPA/DHA (the Omega-3 fatty acid found in fish oils).

! Make sure you buy only high-quality fish oils (EPA/DHA) from which heavy metals, including mercury and lead, have been filtered out.

Proanthocyanidins – part of the powerful flavonoid family

Description: The proanthocyanidins, also known as oligomeric proanthocyanidins (or the OPCs), are part of a 4000-strong family of phytonutrients called the flavonoids, and they're found in grapeseed extract and a pine bark extract called pycnogenol. The OPCs are potent antioxidants. In fact, research shows that their antioxidant activity is fifty times more potent than that of vitamin E, and twenty times greater than that of vitamin C. What's more, they protect vitamins E and C in the skin from being overwhelmed by free radicals.

Grapeseed extracts contain 92 to 95 per cent proanthocyanidins. Pine bark extracts contain 80 to 85 per cent proanthocyanidins.

Skin beauty benefits: The flavonoids (which also includes the polyphenols — think green tea) all have powerful antioxidant properties, but both grapeseed extract and pine bark extract seem to have the best effect on skin and offer greatest protection against premature ageing. They are also great for preserving the youthful resilience and bounce of your skin. OPCs protect capillary walls and promote normal permeability of capillaries. When circulation is enhanced, your skin cells are better nourished. The removal of toxins and waste products from the dermis and epidermis speeds up too. The OPCs have also been shown to improve blood and oxygen flow by dilating blood vessels. Poor skin circulation can lead to water retention, which in turn can cause puffiness around your eyelids.

Research has found that the OPCs strongly inhibit several enzymes involved in the degradation of collagen, elastin and hyaluronic acid. Additionally, OPCs work by protecting and strengthening collagen and elastin and in doing so can help prevent premature ageing.

Proanthocyanidins also help protect against UVB rays. Known as sunburn radiation, UVB light penetrates the epidermis and cripples your skin's natural antioxidant defence system, rendering it virtually powerless against skin-damaging free radicals. Studies have shown that pycnogenol, in particular, reduces skin-cell damage caused by UVB radiation and scavenges the free radicals it generates. Pycnogenol is also an anti-inflammatory agent. Whenever you can reduce inflammation in the skin, free radicals stay in check.

Recommended daily beauty dosage: 50–150mg of OPCs daily. For the treatment of varicose veins and swelling following injury, the dosages range from 150 to 300mg daily.

Beautifying minerals

One way or another, every mineral, like every vitamin, has a part to play in ensuring the health of your skin and in preserving its youth. Balanced ratios are the key when it comes to minerals and their beauty benefits. Each mineral is dependant on another, so if one mineral is out of balance, then all of the others are affected. Four minerals stand out for their role in cultivating healthy, resilient skin cells: zinc, sulphur, silica and selenium. A whole array of other minerals such as iodine, calcium, magnesium and copper are also vital for great skin.

Zinc — a fine beauty mineral

Skin beauty benefits: Zinc helps regenerate skin cells, reduces inflammation, aids in wound healing and is a must in the formation of collagen. Along with supple skin, zinc plays a vital role in strong nails and vibrant hair. Your skin actually contains about twenty per cent of your body's zinc. Without enough zinc and B6, stretch marks readily appear and the skin sags and wrinkles easily. Zinc promotes cell growth, boosts immunity and helps treat acne when combined with vitamins A and B. It is also necessary in the treatment of eczema and psoriasis, and it aids in the absorption of many other vitamins and minerals. It's needed for oil gland function and local skin hormone activation too. The absorption of zinc can be impeded by birth control pills, high levels of copper, oestrogen replacement therapy and excessive alcohol consumption.

Deficiency symptoms: Slow healing, dandruff, lowered resistance to infections.

Recommend daily beauty dosage: 15–30mg (zinc picolinate).

Sulphur — skin smoother & beauty mineral extraordinaire

Skin beauty benefits: This beauty mineral — housed in every cell of the body — plays a vital role in building tissue and enhancing the health of your cells. It regulates the sodium–potassium balance, bringing oxygen and nutrients to your cells and neutralising wastes. It also helps give sheen and gloss to your hair and strength to your nails. The keratin in your epidermis as well as your fingernails and hair is especially rich in sulphur.

The best source of sulphur is methyl-sulphonyl-methane, or MSM. It's a superb free radical scavenger, plus it also slows down the loss of collagen, stabilises connective tissue and even helps regulate the way insulin behaves in the body. MSM is extremely water-soluble, so it is destroyed by cooking, and it diminishes with age.

Recommended daily beauty dosage: 2000mg of MSM.

Deficiency symptoms: Dry scalp, rashes, eczema, weak hair and nails, scaly skin.

Selenium — super-antioxidant mineral

Skin beauty benefits: Selenium boosts your body's production of glutathione peroxidase, a potent antioxidant enzyme. Like the other antioxidants, selenium helps to preserve tissue elasticity because of its ability to slow down oxidation of polyunsaturated fatty acids, which can bring about cross-linking and cause skin to sag and lose its tone. It also aids in the synthesis of certain prostaglandin hormones that affect the smoothness and texture of the skin. Plus, selenium halts inflammation and aids in removing toxins. It also helps give your tissues elasticity and is an important factor in the prevention of premature ageing in the skin. Selenium has been shown to help fade liver spots!

Recommended daily beauty dosage: 25 micrograms (mcg) selenium (selenomethione, which is the natural organic form of selenium). It's interesting to note that the recommended dosages in the United States range from 200 to 400 micrograms (mcg) daily!

Deficiency symptoms: Premature ageing, growth impairment, muscle degeneration.

Silica – the beauty mineral

Skin beauty benefits: Silica is an essential mineral for health and beauty. It strengthens collagen and elastin fibres and contributes to tissue elasticity. It also aids in collagen formation, keeps skin taut, strengthens bones and skin tissues and helps prevent wrinkles. Silica creates strong shiny hair and holds moisture in your skin, making it plump and smooth. The highest concentration of silica (silicon dioxide) is found in connective tissues, cartilage and your skin.

Recommended daily beauty dosage: 20–30mg.

Deficiency symptoms: Premature wrinkles, lack of skin tone, sagging skin and brittle nails.

Copper

Skin beauty benefits: You've probably noticed copper in a number of moisturisers these days. Copper is involved in collagen and elastin production and as well as the production of the moisture-holding molecules glycosaminoglycans (or GAGs for short). It also helps synthesise superoxide dismutase (SOD), an antioxidant enzyme that's very active in your skin, and it detoxifies oxygen radicals. Copper is found in a variety of foods and a copper deficiency is uncommon except in people taking high doses of zinc supplements.

Beauty sources: Almonds, beans, crab, mushrooms, oysters, pecans, prunes, sunflower seeds, whole grains.

Beautifying vitamins

Although vitamins are needed in relatively small amounts, they are absolutely essential to create new cells and keep your skin looking youthful and fresh. However, most of them can't be manufactured by your body on its own; they must be obtained from food or through dietary supplements. Some vitamins, such as vitamin A, C and E, act as antioxidants.

The beauty-promoting B vitamins

Description: The B vitamins are a group that includes vitamins B1 (thiamine), B2 (riboflavin), B3 (niacin), B5 (pantothenate), B6 (pyridoxine), B12 (cyancobalamine), folate (B9), PABA, inositol, biotin and choline. The Bs are water soluble and grouped together as a complex because, when naturally occurring, they are always found together.

Skin beauty benefits: The B vitamins play a pivotal role in maintaining healthy skin. They help rebuild and repair skin tissue, and they also generate the energy needed to keep cells working and help oxygenate the skin. They are often called the anti-stress vitamins. The Bs also naturally help to prevent premature ageing and acne, as well as promoting healthy circulation and metabolism. They are essential for wound healing (sunburn, bruises, infections), aiding new cell growth and increasing vitality. Remember that, as they're part of a synergistic family that work best as a team, they should all be taken together.

Outstanding sources: Lean beef, chicken, egg yolks, liver, milk, brewer's yeast, whole grains, alfalfa, almonds, sunflower seeds, soy products, green leafy vegetables, blue–green algae, fresh wheat germ, molasses, peas and beans.

Deficiency symptoms: Sore mouth and lips, eczema, skin lesions, dandruff, pale complexion, pigmentation problems, premature wrinkles. Lack of B vitamins can also cause dry and cracking lips.

✔ Stress, alcohol and the contraceptive pill also increase the need for the B vitamins.

Ensure that your multi-vitamin/mineral nutrient contains ample amounts of each of the Bs. Adults should take 50 to 100mg per day of each of the B vitamins, except for B12, which should not exceed 1mg (1000 micrograms) per day. Just about every mineral is also needed in a balanced ratio for your skin to look and perform its best. So make sure you choose an excellent multi nutrient regime with a balanced ratio of all the minerals and vitamins.

Pro-beauty probiotics – feed your good bugs

For gorgeous skin it's absolutely imperative to have an abundance of friendly intestinal flora. The big problem is that our modern lifestyle poses a challenge to the good bacteria that live in our gut. From the antibiotics we take, to our diet, to the chlorinated water we drink and shower in, our lives are full of threats to the survival of our good bugs. And when the good bugs start to lose the battle, more virulent bad bugs, like the *Candida albicans* strain, which occur naturally, can take over. This can contribute to an imbalance of good and bad bacteria in the gut and even in the skin, which can set the stage for various skin conditions as well as a whole host of other health problems. During the Grogeous Skin program, I recommend that you feed your good bugs every day with probiotics, for optimal digestion, and health.

'Beneficial bacteria' like *acidophilus* and *bifidus* can help with a whole range of problems, including acne, poor digestion, itchy skin, eczema, dandruff, athlete's foot, allergies, sinus and vaginal yeast issues. But note that these factors can be symptoms of a more serious syndrome that often includes autoimmune diseases, nutritional deficiencies and food sensitivities.

Simple solutions to good gut ecology

- Take a good probiotic, which you'll find at a good health-food store. See Resources, page 306, for details.
- Eat plain yoghurt and drink kefir (always unsweetened, though, as the 'bad' bugs thrive on sugar; they also thrive on flour and starch).
- Eat lots of garlic, which kills yeast and just about any other bacteria.

See Chapter 8 for the recommended dosages and supplements for your 30-day Gorgeous Skin plan.

5

The Protectors

Three Keys to Slowing the Ageing Clock

'Exuberance is Beauty.'
— William Blake

Contrary to what many skincare companies would love you to believe, your ageing clock is set from within. And no matter how fantastic a cream or serum is made to sound, it can't turn back the clock. In this chapter, we'll be discussing the third tier of the prevention program: the three 'protectors' that play an extremely important role in your natural anti-ageing strategy. Even if you follow the Gorgeous Skin diet to a T and avoid excessive sun and cigarette smoke, unless you implement the following 'protectors' you will be compromising an optimum result. The protectors are:

- a relaxation method
- adequate sleep
- moderate exercise.

Each of these has a profound impact on your hormonal system and on reducing free radical activity, thereby greatly improving how your skin looks and ages. A big part of ageing — along with cumulative free radical damage, genetic, and environmental factors — is that, as you get older, the production of hormones that made you bloom as an adolescent begins to slow down. A lot of these changes occur in your thirties, but you often don't see the effects until your mid-forties. So anything you can do to safeguard your delicate hormonal balance will improve how you and your skin age.

Relaxation — de-stressing the skin

Countless studies show that people who do some form of deep relaxation such as yoga or meditation look younger and are biologically younger than those who don't! This is because deep relaxation can help switch on your body's calming nervous system, which ultimately leads to a shift from the production of age-promoting stress hormones to calming, age-protecting ones. You may think there is no way you can find time to meditate or practise yoga — let alone get enough sleep — but the payoffs are so enormous that I encourage you to make the time, especially during the 30-day program. By incorporating the protectors into your daily routine, you'll be on your way to achieving a radiant glow and lasting youthfulness. So up your relaxation ante!

Long-term unresolved stress can wreak havoc on your appearance and accelerate ageing. And when you consider that your skin is your largest organ, it's not surprising that stress manifests itself in the way you look. We've all seen the change in someone's appearance after they've been through an unpleasant divorce or the death of a close relative. But you'd be surprised at how much of an impact chronic everyday stress has on your skin.

As will be discussed in Chapter 6, when your body is under stress it releases a number of stress hormones such as adrenaline, noradrenaline and cortisol — a response that's valuable for enduring short-term stressful situations but destructive if sustained over longer periods of time. The prolonged flood of stress hormones results in long-term changes in your skin and hair. Your body redirects critical nutrients from your skin to vital organs (such as your heart, brain and lungs) and over time this process deprives your skin of oxygen and nourishment, resulting in less-than-gorgeous skin. Extended periods of stress also affect your metabolic functions by slowing down the renewal of your skin cells, leading to dull, sallow skin. Stress also upsets your body's fluid balance, which can make your skin sag and look dehydrated.

When you're under pressure, you also tend to tighten your muscles, and this restricts blood flow to your skin cells. At the same time, it slows down the lymphatic drainage into and out of every organ so that your cells can't defend themselves from infection. You may then notice you have dull, sallow skin that is prone to spots, strange bumps, and allergic reactions and chapped lips that are susceptible to sores. The stress response also amplifies free radical production, which accelerates ageing even further.

Stress — no matter what kind or where it comes from — can have adverse effects on the normal production of your hormones. Under increased stress your body will make more cortisol in order to cope. Your hormone-making pathway (steroidogenic pathway) that creates cortisol is the same pathway that makes your 'sex hormones' (oestrogen, progesterone and testosterone). So in effect, under stress, your body makes more cortisol at the expense of your sex hormones. Remember, all of your hormones, especially adequate amounts of oestrogen, are required for the production of collagen and the moisture factor hyaluronic acid, which keeps your skin moist and plump. So you need to manage stress in order to preserve your skin and keep it in peak condition.

It's only recently that we've begun to appreciate the intimate physiological relationship between our neural (nervous system) and dermal (skin) systems. Your epidermis (the outer most layer of your skin) and the prenatal brain originate from the same region in an embryo. There are immune cells that reside beneath our skin, and these cells have their own nerve supply. When we feel stressed, the brain sends a message to the pituitary, adrenal and sex glands. Certain hormones are produced that flood the skin surface with oils, priming it for acne. At the same time, inflammatory mediators are released to the surface, triggering itchiness or the symptoms of conditions like psoriasis. The stress hormones can also cause inflammation that impedes your skin's ability to renew itself and weakens its defences against environmental damage.

New studies suggest that stress also depletes your skin's barrier of moisture, making it vulnerable to a host of non-specific ills. A study with the University of California in San Francisco showed that women undergoing a divorce have a weaker moisture barrier than those who are happily married.[41]

At this point just in case you're thinking that you probably don't encounter enough stress to have an impact on your skin, think again! Today, the pace of life has become so feverish, the opportunities for rest and recuperation so restricted, that a whole heap of everyday hassles have been redefined as stressful: your child's party entertainer cancels on short notice; ten important e-mails arrive on your screen simultaneously; your laptop crashes; your mobile phone suddenly conks out; your kids walk in and demand dinner!

Remember, stress isn't all bad. A challenging life mobilises our bodies to promote adaptation and it actually improves memory, immune function and metabolism. It's just the wear and tear from a bad lifestyle, from sleep deprivation and from continued tension and anxiety, and from a lack of control over our lives, that can cause long-term problems. It's really our response to stress that matters. A change of mindset is what's required, rather than a change of circumstance. If you can deal with stress in a positive, constructive way and manage the emotions and habits that create stress — and, ultimately, ageing — your endocrine system will function optimally and it will help keep your skin in great shape.

So remember, a major key to gorgeous skin is keeping stress levels in check and sticking to a daily relaxation program. When you're relaxed your superficial circulation increases, cortisol levels stay low, your hormone output improves, especially the hormones that control healing and cell replication, and you benefit from more endorphins, the hormones that create the 'feel-good' factor. Yoga, meditation, moderate exercise and deep breathing are some of the most powerful ways to create beautiful skin from within.

Meditation

People who meditate regularly actually look younger and are biologically younger than people who don't. In fact, studies have found that, on average, long-term meditators show biological ages almost twelve years younger than their chronological ages![42] Other studies have shown that certain hormonal changes usually associated with ageing can be slowed or reversed through regular meditation.[43] It's one of the most powerful anti-ageing tools you have at your disposal.

Despite the good sense of it and the overwhelming benefits, some people are still resistant to meditation. For many, meditation still conjures up images of incense and chanting and sitting still for hours with your legs twisted like a pretzel. But the truth is: meditation can be whatever you want it to be, as long as it allows your mind some quiet time and your nervous system to switch into a relaxed, anti-ageing mode.

A growing number of Australians say they practise some form of meditation regularly. Meditation classes today are filled by mainstream people who don't own crystals, don't subscribe to New Age magazines, and don't even reside in Byron Bay or Nimbin! Meditation isn't religious; it isn't even necessarily spiritual. It crosses all spiritual, financial and socio-economic boundaries. The benefits are vast — and, short of potentially dangerous shots of human growth hormone, it's one of the most amazing things you can do for your health and, of course, your skin.

What meditation can do for you

We live such fast-paced lives we're often in 'sympathetic overdrive' mode, where our adrenal glands constantly pump out cortisol and adrenaline, which is the body's 'stress' response. During meditation you switch into a deep anti-ageing, relaxation mode, whereby your body reduces its oxygen consumption, your breath rate slows, and your levels of blood lactate decrease (high lactate levels are associated with uneasiness and anxiety and low levels with peace and calm). Your adrenal glands also produce less adrenaline and noradrenaline and pump out less age-accelerating cortisol.

At the University of Wisconsin at Madison in the United States, researcher Richard Davidson used brain imaging to show that meditation shifts activity in the prefrontal cortex (right behind your forehead) from the right hemisphere to the left. People who have a negative disposition tend to be right-prefrontal oriented; left-prefrontals have more enthusiasm and more interests, relax more and tend to be happier. Davidson's research also suggests that, through regular meditation, the brain is reoriented from a stressful fight-or-flight mode to one of acceptance, a shift that increases contentment and happiness.[44]

Other studies have found that regular meditation increases production of the hormone DHEA, which drops off considerably with age, causing countless problems.[45] DHEA is vital in maintaining a good mood, normal sex drive, stable body fat ratio and a high level of energy. DHEA also boosts our immune system and brain, helps us to handle stress, aids in normalising our blood lipid (fat) profiles and protects our heart. In a young, healthy body, DHEA is converted to oestrogen and testosterone along with other sex hormones, providing the benefits of *all these* hormones.

In addition, DHEA protects against the ravages of the stress hormone cortisol, which, when elevated, can lead to memory loss,

Oestrogen and ageing

Oestrogen, without a doubt, is one of the hormones that keeps women's skin youthful and resilient. It's responsible for the depositing of fat under the skin, giving rise to the soft and fine-textured skin that many women enjoy during their younger years. It also causes fluid and salt retention in our tissues, which helps plump up and fill out the skin. During the reproductive years, a woman's body produces enough oestrogen to support the structure of her skin, but she loses much of this as she goes through menopause, when oestrogen levels drop significantly. This loss of oestrogen is also commonly accompanied by a loss of collagen, making the skin thinner, drier and more prone to wrinkling.

There is no doubt that a loss of oestrogen is detrimental to the appearance and texture of skin. Even though there's a good deal of research showing that taking hormone replacement therapy or HRT (specifically oestrogen) improves the appearance and texture of the skin, recent research has revealed that the potential problems of HRT can far outweigh their benefits. I highly recommend finding a doctor or other qualified health practitioner who specialises in natural hormone therapy and natural hormone replacement.

Unbalanced stress in your life also causes your hypothalamus, a gland considered by many doctors to be the 'brain's brain', to decline in function. As your hypothalamus deteriorates, it becomes far less adept at responding to minor imbalances. Sometimes it calls for the production of too few hormones and sometimes too many. In effect, it loses its elasticity and flexibility. This degeneration triggers the dysfunction of the rest of your endocrine system. Fat clings to the abdomen. Memories fade. Viruses go unopposed. Eye muscles lose their focus. Immunity wanes. Sex drive declines. Ageing runs rampant. Skin loses its suppleness.

Enter meditation. If done regularly, meditation can help increase your DHEA levels.

TIP

Optimism reduces cortisol levels, so make fun a priority and practise having a positive attitude, even in the midst of a crisis!

accelerated ageing, and a general decline in immunity. When cortisol levels rise at the expense of DHEA, an imbalance arises in your DHEA/cortisol ratio, which is considered to be a key to the biochemistry of accelerated ageing. Chronically high cortisol and low DHEA levels are found in nearly every major illness and in accelerated ageing. High DHEA, on the other hand, promotes the healthy maintenance and regeneration of your body's systems and is believed to counter the effects of the ageing process.

Production of DHEA in turn causes your pituitary gland to release more of the anti-ageing growth hormone HGH, which has a powerful impact on how your skin looks and ages. Many researchers believe that one of the primary reasons we go downhill as we age is the deterioration of our endocrine system, the producer of important hormones such as HGH, which repairs your muscles and tissues, builds your immunity and helps keep your skin youthful and gorgeous.

This is why meditation is so powerful; it activates your body's own natural anti-ageing healing force and boosts your hormonal system. Research indicates that people who meditate regularly achieve a marked reduction in their oxygen use (this means less destructive free radicals are produced) and have a notably lower secretion of stress hormones, an increase in immune factors, improved hormone function and calm brainwave activity, all of which indicate a slowing of the ageing process.

In one study on meditation, researchers measured biological age (how old a person is physiologically rather than chronologically), determinants of blood pressure, vision and hearing.[46] All these factors were improved with meditation. Participants practising meditation for five years were physiologically twelve years younger than their non-meditating counterparts![47] Even the short-term participants were physiologically five years younger than the controls. One reason among many to get meditating!

Transcendental meditation

The most extensively researched form of meditation is transcendental meditation (TM). The TM technique doesn't require specific beliefs or the adoption of a particular lifestyle. In TM you repeat a mantra over and over, which is a Sanskrit (the classic language of India) syllable; it's easy and doesn't require any special ability. People throughout the world of all ages, educational backgrounds, cultures, and religions practise the technique and enjoy its wide range of benefits.

Over five hundred scientific studies have been conducted on the physiological, psychological and sociological effects of TM, and these studies have been carried out at 210 different universities and research institutions in more than thirty countries. Results of the studies have appeared in more than a hundred journals, including major scientific journals. In 1967, Dr Herbert Benson, a professor of medicine at Harvard Medical School, found that when a group of TM practitioners meditated they used seventeen per cent less oxygen, lowered their heart rates by three beats a minute and increased their theta brainwave — the one that comes just before sleep — without slipping into the brainwave pattern of actual sleep.

Studies show that regular practise of TM is highly beneficial and leads to:

- reduced stress: the deep rest that the mind and body get in TM eliminates mental and physical stress and fatigue
- increased intelligence: the mind returns to its natural state of alertness and in turn this increases a person's intelligence level
- increased creativity: TM practitioners become more creative than others because the mind is in a refreshed and relaxed state
- improved memory: the mind's state of alertness increases its capacity for memorisation
- improved health: incidence of illness and risk of heart disease is reduced significantly among meditators
- reduced high blood pressure: free from stress and anxiety, there is a lower incidence of high blood pressure
- increased energy: with better health and mental state, TM practitioners are always full of energy
- reduced insomnia: being relieved of stress and anxiety, followers of TM experience better and healthier sleep patterns
- reversal of biological ageing: those practising TM are, on average, biologically five to twelve years younger!
- increased happiness: meditators have warmer interpersonal relationships, less anxiety, increased self-esteem and self-confidence, increased problem-solving ability, and greater creativity, all of which bring more happiness to their lives.

In your jam-packed schedule it's probably hard to imagine slowing down on a regular basis, even for ten minutes, but I can't emphasise just how important it is for your health (and specifically your skin) to do so. Along with your diet — and, of course, avoiding excessive sun — meditation is one of the most important things you can do for your skin and health.

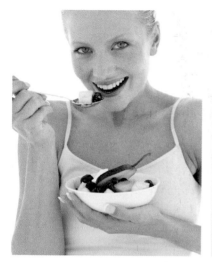
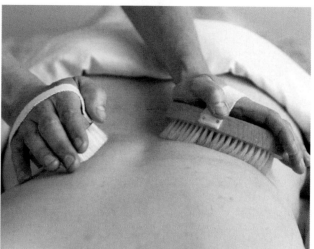
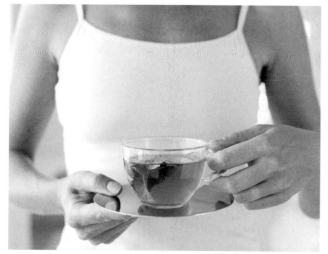
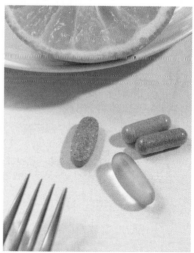

build beauty from within

Cleanse your body with detoxifying foods and plenty of good liquids,
stimulate your lymphatic system with skin brushing
and supplement your diet with skin rejuvenating nutrients.

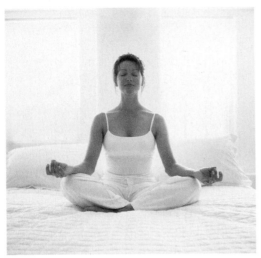

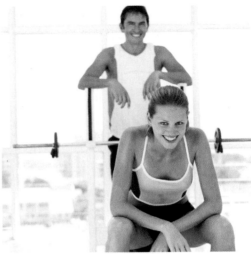

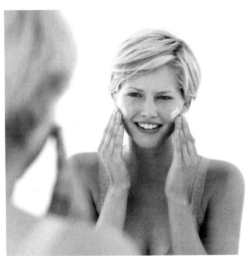

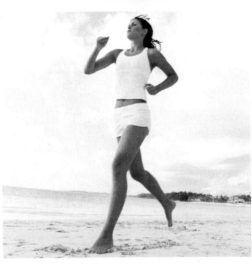

relax, energise and protect

Switch on your calming nervous system with yoga, increase your muscle mass with moderate weight training, stimulate your blood flow with aerobic exercise, and protect yourself from the skin ageing UV rays.

So how do I meditate?

Learning to meditate doesn't have to be complicated. Find a quiet space free from distractions and either sit or lie down on a comfortable mat, bed, cushion or chair. Relax every muscle in your body from bottom to top, close your eyes and breathe deeply. On page 116 I've included a sample of a basic meditation session to give you a starting point, but I encourage you to find a style that's right for you. There are some great guided meditations on DVDs, CDs and tapes, too.

Even if you've tried to meditate and given up because of all of the thoughts racing through your head, try again. Some people believe that this is an important aspect of meditation, because it allows you to release all of these thoughts from your subconscious mind into your conscious mind. You can think of it as sorting out the clutter hidden in your attic or defragmenting your computer! Learning how to quieten your mind and actually allowing yourself to slow down isn't going to happen overnight.

To help pause your internal dialogue, silently repeat a word or a mantra. It can be religious or philosophical or just a calming sound, as long as it makes you feel good. Or just focus on your breathing. When thoughts intrude, don't let it worry you — just start again. The most important things to focus on are breathing easily and consistently and not reacting to outside thoughts. You might need several tries before you slip into a tranquil state, but any amount of time where you are quiet and still will benefit your health.

Commit yourself to twenty minutes a day for meditation. You can look at your watch on occasion but don't set an alarm, as it may give you a fright and ruin your relaxation. After you finish, sit quietly for a couple of minutes and try to carry your calm, anti-ageing, meditative attitude into your daily life. Your mind will be clearer, you'll be able to perform daily tasks more efficiently, you'll feel rejuvenated and refreshed, and you'll be slowing your ageing clock.

Basic meditation session

- Find a quiet place away from all noise and telephones (that means your mobile phone too).
- Sit in a comfortable place (or lie down if you can stay awake!).
- Straighten your spine, elongate your neck, and lower your chin a bit towards your chest.
- Spend the first few minutes relaxing every muscle in your body from your toes to your head. Focus on smooth, easy breathing through your nose.
- As you breathe, concentrate on each inhalation, exhalation, and the natural pauses that occur in between.
- If you begin to lose focus and think about other things, visualise your thoughts as clouds that come into your mind and gently disperse.
- At the end of your session, be sure to move slowly for the next couple of minutes, especially if you've been lying down.

Yoga

If you're really serious and you want to turn back the clock, try yoga. Yoga cultivates calm by driving down levels of stress hormones that create havoc for your general health and that of your skin. Plus, the beauty benefits are endless. Through breathing techniques (*pranayama*) and physical postures (*asanas*), yoga increases circulation and brings much-needed nutrients and oxygen to rejuvenate and revitalise your skin; it switches on your anti-ageing parasympathetic (calming) nervous system which has both mental and physical benefits; it can soften facial wrinkles and produces a natural face lift through inverted postures; it encourages proper circulation of blood and lymph fluid, enhances digestion, strengthens the hormonal system and lubricates joints. Several of the postures also provide a gentle massage to your internal organs, stimulating them to gradually release toxins. When you stimulate your lymphatic system your body can get rid of toxins more efficiently, which ultimately means clearer skin. Yoga will also help you sleep a lot better.

Another beauty bonus is that the inverted yoga postures can increase blood supply to the hair follicles in your scalp, which may delay the onset of grey hair. Plus, the improved nourishment of the hair follicles creates thicker, healthier hair. Increased flexibility of the neck produced by the different yoga postures also helps by removing the pressure on the blood vessels and nerves in your neck, therefore further enhancing the blood supply to your scalp.

Sleep easy

A study from the Defence Institute of Physiology and Allied Sciences in Dehli, India, showed that three months of twice-daily hour-long Hatha yoga sessions helps alleviate insomnia by stimulating the production of melatonin.[48]

Yoga isn't just a great form of relaxation, it can also be a great form of exercise. There are many different types of yoga. Some, like Hatha, are very relaxing, while others, like Ashtanga, Iyengar and Bikram, are more vigorous. The key to taking years from your face and adding years to your life is finding a style that you enjoy and sticking to it. If yoga isn't your thing, Tai Chi and Qi Gong are great ways to switch on your calming nervous system and help slow the ageing process.

Three yoga postures (*asanas*)

These three poses are gentle and effective but they're best not practised in isolation. If you haven't done yoga before, attend a few classes and ask your teacher to make sure you're aligned properly.

Child's Pose (*Balasana*)

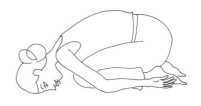

The Child's Pose is particularly good for relieving stress and fatigue. It's also believed to calm the brain and gently stretch the hips, ankles and thighs.

Start by kneeling on a mat on the floor. Then put your feet together, making sure your big toes are touching, and sit on your heels. Then separate your knees so they are about as wide as your hips. Exhale and lay your body (torso) between your thighs. Lengthen your tailbone away from the back of your pelvis while you lift the base of your skull away from the back of your neck.

Then lay your hands on the floor alongside your body, palms up, and release the fronts of your shoulders towards the floor. You should feel how the weight of the front shoulders pulls the shoulder blades wide across your back.

The Child's pose is a resting pose, so you can stay in this pose anywhere from 30 seconds to a few minutes, breathing naturally and deeply.

The Cat Pose (*Bidalasana*)

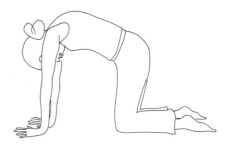

This pose is wonderful for stretching the spine, including the middle to upper back along with the shoulders. The Cat Pose is also believed to stimulate spinal fluid and the digestive tract.

Start on all fours with your back flat, hands beneath your shoulders and knees directly below your hips. Make sure your hands are fully spread, with your middle fingers pointing straight ahead. Inhaling, arch your back, moving your chest and head forward and up. As you exhale, slowly tuck in your tailbone and round your back like an angry cat. Repeat 5 times slowly.

Downward-facing Dog (*Adho Mukha Svanasana*)

The Downward-facing Dog can help increase blood flow to the facial skin. It's also good for relieving stress and calming the brain. This pose is also great for stretching the shoulders, calves and hamstrings and it's believed to improve digestion and energise the body.

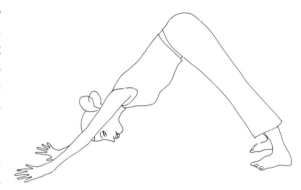

Start by coming onto the mat on your hands and knees. Kneel and place your hands on the ground in front of your knees and spread your fingers wide. Step both feet back, one at a time, and gently straighten your legs, but make sure you don't lock your knees. With your feet hip-width apart, inhale and raise your buttocks and hips. Lower your head towards the floor, relax your neck and lift shoulders back. Release your chest through your shoulders and work your heels to the ground. Breathe deeply.

The Downward-facing Dog is one of the poses in the traditional Sun Salutation sequence. It's also an excellent *yoga asana* (pose) on its own. Stay in this pose anywhere from one to three minutes and make sure you breathe naturally and deeply. Come out of the pose by bending your knees gently to the floor, then rest in Child's Pose.

NOTE: Any of the inverted yoga positions increases blood flow to the facial skin.

The mystery of beauty

We all tend to focus far too much on how we look rather than how we feel. Our minds and souls need as much attention as our face and bodies! Both yoga and mediation create inner focus and calm. Some of the most attractive people have an internal brilliance — their eyes are bright and often sparkle, their skin has a subtle glow, they radiate an inner beauty which has nothing to do with their clothes, their weight or even their bone structure. It's an internal light that shines from within. For a physically attractive woman to be beautiful, the inside must match the outside!

Beauty is not in the face,
Beauty is a light in the heart.
— Kahlil Gibran (1883–1931)

Deep breathing

Air is the most vital nutrient for your body. You can survive for weeks without food, days without water, and only minutes without air. Yet most people only tend to breathe very shallowly. In fact, most of us use only about twenty per cent of our lung capacity.

Rapid, shallow breathing is a common involuntary reaction and is part of your natural stress response. When you breathe shallowly, the stale air in the lower part of your lungs isn't fully expelled and when you inhale, your lungs don't fill up beyond the upper third of their actual volume. Then, carbon dioxide isn't properly removed from your blood, and consequently your brain, nervous system and skin aren't fully oxygenated. In essence, you are using a fraction of your vital capacity, creating an inefficient oxygen exchange in your bloodstream that robs the skin of its vitality and glow. How does this lack of oxygen affect us? It actually causes us to make more free radicals.

Seventy per cent of elimination from your body is done through breathing! Imagine how your skin would look if you practised deep breathing! Think about how your skin glows after a relaxing walk in the country. This is because as you naturally relax and exert yourself, your breathing gets deeper and slower, bringing more oxygen to your skin.

Yoga and meditation are great tools to get you breathing deeply.

The force of your breath and the rhythmic pressure changes in your chest also pump your lymphatic circulation, which helps detoxify your blood. Anything you can do to increase oxygen to your skin will make your skin glow. Much of this radiance is due to the efficient elimination of toxins and waste, plus the increased flow of oxygen-rich blood to your face. Improving circulation and oxygen flow can help to slow the ageing process.

Now here's a fun addition to your anti-ageing protectors — sex! A study conducted by the Royal Edinburgh Hospital in Scotland found that people who have sex at least three times per week on average tend to look ten or more years younger that their real ages![49] The researchers suggest that the sex triggers the release of growth hormone, which promotes lean muscle and contributes to maintaining a youthful appearance. Sex also increases the amount of oestrogen and endorphins in your body, making your hair, eyes and skin more vibrant. Plus it dilates arteries, sending blood to the surface of your skin, giving you the telltale glow. The increased heart rate and deep breathing accounts for the improvement in circulation. As the fresh blood supply arrives, your cells, organs and muscles are saturated with fresh oxygen and hormones. You also radiate an energy that makes you look more alive and beautiful, too!

Pranayama yoga breathing for radiant skin

Sit in a comfortable position. Open your chest by pulling your shoulder blades together. Let your chest expand as you inhale slowly through your nose, and let it flatten out naturally as you exhale through your mouth. Do this for a few minutes every morning to help give your skin a gorgeous, radiant glow for the day.

Beauty sleep

One of the best ways to stay young may be to get some serious shut-eye. Sleep replenishes, rejuvenates and restores. The skin's rate of cell renewal (a function essential for fresh, young-looking skin) is at its highest when we sleep. So you just can't expect to skip sleep and have radiantly skin. A chronic lack of sleep will take its toll on your complexion. Yet forty per cent of Australians have suffered insomnia at some point and don't get enough sleep. When you sleep, your body goes into repair mode: toxins are removed, immune system cells are activated and hormones go to work. With chronic sleep deprivation, your body's ability to heal itself is interrupted, which can lead to emotional and physical problems, including premature ageing. A recent study at the University of Chicago found that the physiological effects of sleep deprivation mimic those of ageing.[50] Sleep deprivation can also cause an impaired ability to regulate glucose and higher than usual levels of cortisol.

 TIP

Don't eat any food that can cause a rapid rise in blood sugar — like biscuits or chocolate — before going to bed. These types of high-GI foods can interfere with growth hormone production, robbing you of its essential anti-ageing action.

It's not enough to get an adequate amount of sleep; you have to get enough of the *right kind* of sleep. This means deep sleep, which helps promote growth hormone release (remember: your youth hormone) and the repair and regeneration which naturally follows this release. During sleep, especially Phase Four deep delta sleep, your body secretes growth hormone and other skin-growth factors that help stimulate the production of collagen and new skin cells. The more deep sleep you get, the more you'll naturally help slow down the ageing process.

Growth hormone isn't the only powerful anti-ageing chemical that you secrete while you sleep. Your pineal gland increases its production of the hormone melatonin (you actually produce five times more melatonin at night than during the day). Melatonin has also been called the 'pacemaker of the ageing clock'! Not only does it assist in sleeping, but it's also an important detoxifier of free radicals, especially the very damaging hydroxyl radical. Dr Denham Harman, the founder of the free radical theory of ageing in 1954, contended that the downward slide begins at age twenty-seven, which means it's never too early to protect against the free radical cascade in your body! But it's never too late to improve on what you've got, either.

How much sleep is enough? The general rule is seven to eight hours every night. Some people need less, others more. The key is restful sleep, which means you drift off easily and sleep soundly through the night, then are alert, refreshed and energetic all day long! If you are sleepy during the day it means you've incurred a sleep debt. Research lasting two weeks found that this sleep debt remains until paid off with extra sleep.[52] You generally don't notice the debt if you're stimulated, drink coffee or are at a time

Sleep and stress

Seratonin and melatonin, hormones that regulate your body's natural 24-hour sleep cycle, are often among the first chemical messengers to fail during times of stress. If they aren't at optimum levels, you'll find it hard to fall asleep, will wake frequently, may have vivid dreams and won't feel rested in the morning.

Cortisol can also interrupt sleep by causing a heightened state of alertness and arousal. If high levels of cortisol are present in your bloodstream at night, getting a good night's sleep becomes almost impossible. A study at the Sleep Research and Treatment Centre of the Pennsylvania State University College of Medicine in the United States found that chronic insomniacs have much higher levels of cortisol than their well-rested counterparts.[51]

Additionally, a decrease in REM sleep appears to be associated with elevated levels of cortisol. Cortisol levels normally peak in the mornings and decline at night, matching a person's sleep patterns, but those with decreased REM sleep appear to have higher cortisol levels at night.

of the day when daytime 'alerting' (the peak of activity in the morning or early evening) banishes the fatigue for a time. It's during the afternoon or while relaxing or doing repetitive tasks (like driving) that the body demands its repayment.

A recent study conducted by the American National Institute of Mental Health found that, if left to their own devices, people slept on average fourteen hours per night![53] Interestingly, the subjects claimed at the end of the three weeks that never before had they known what it felt like to be fully rested and awake!

Sleeping for fourteen hours isn't exactly practical and realistic in today's world, but if you always need an alarm clock to wake up, you probably aren't getting enough sleep. How can you tell if you are not getting enough sleep? Obviously, if you don't feel rested in the morning, you're not getting enough quality sleep. If you feel drowsy during the day, you probably need more sleep. You may have to evaluate your lifestyle and make some changes. When people are busy and crowd their schedules with activities, sleep often gets put aside. If you are serious about gorgeous skin, it's essential that you schedule at least seven to eight hours of deep, restful sleep per night.

If you're under a lot of stress and find it difficult to switch off your mind, consider meditating before sleep or doing some form of relaxation such as deep breathing or self-hypnosis. Take a warm bath, add a few drops of lavender essential oil, and drink some relaxing herbal tea, such as chamomile, passionflower, valerian root, hops, skullcap or a combination of these. The minerals calcium and magnesium also work well to help you get the deep sleep your body needs to keep your skin gorgeous and youthful.

Along with the herbs mentioned above there are two different classes of natural supplements that can help promote sleep: melatonin and 5-HTP.

Melatonin production drops off sharply over the age of forty. So it's generally recommended for people over forty and also for night workers, people travelling across time zones, those with high levels of cortisol, and women with hot flushes. It is not recommended for people with autoimmune disease.

! Consult your health professional before supplementing with
melatonin.

5-HTP is another great natural sleep inducer. It's also an anti-depres-
sant, anti-anxiety supplement, and tends to curb carbohydrate and
chocolate cravings. If your depression is strongly related to poor and
difficult sleep, 5-HTP should be considered.

Since sleep is so important for rejuvenation, it's essential that you
do everything possible to enhance your sleep experience. But forgo
alcohol before sleep! A few drinks may make you feel sleepy, but
they will inevitably lead to a poor night's sleep. You'll most likely
fall asleep easily but you'll probably wake a few hours later. This is
because alcohol causes the release of noradrenaline — a hormone
that increases as a result of stress or excitement. So hours after a
drink a burst of noradrenaline can occur and bring you back to con-
sciousness, ruining a good night's sleep.

Wake up to wellness

In our accelerated society we have been programmed to believe that
the best part of waking up is the coffee in our cup. But there is nothing healthful or anti-ageing about coffee, especially first thing in the
morning on an empty stomach! In fact, all it does is give us a stimulating rush so we can jump right back into the stress cycle.

Just 400 or so grams of your favourite coffee contains enough caffeine to more than double your adrenaline level. Pump out enough
adrenaline and your cortisol levels rise. In fact, three cups of coffee
a day can cause your blood cortisol levels to stay high for about
eighteen hours a day, as opposed to the usual few hours for which
cortisol is supposed to be elevated!

Instead of coffee, start the day with herbal tea, deep breathing, stretching, yoga, meditation or a walk. Bring balance to your endocrine system and strength to your nervous system so that you can set your mind and body right to enjoy a great day.

Exercise — the great anti-ager

A regular exercise program is another key component to the fountain of youth. Regular, moderate exercise plays a crucial role in keeping your skin young. It stimulates your circulatory system so nutrient-rich blood can access more areas of your body. It also improves cell nutrition, especially to the dermal layers of your skin, enhances and accelerates healing, and can boost your anti-ageing hormones. But be careful. Excessive exercise can actually accelerate ageing! Burning more than about 12,500 kilojoules a week through aerobic exercise tends to be 'pro-ageing' and to generate oxidative free radicals, which, over the long term, can age your cells more.

In our twenties, our bodies slow down production of many of our hormones by about 10 per cent each decade. By the age of sixty-five we are making only 15 to 20 per cent of the amount of HGH that we made when we were in our twenties. I'm sure you can see why injections of HGH are such a popular anti-ageing treatment but you can increase your supply of growth hormone just by working out, especially through weight training. When your lean muscle mass increases, the levels of your sex hormones and steroid hormones — which preserve water balance and the youthful appearance of skin — increase in direct proportion to the increase in your muscle mass.

HGH is secreted in bursts during the day, but its prime activity takes place during the early hours of deep sleep. It isn't called beauty sleep for nothing! Regular exercise is a great way to increase HGH. But for best results, don't eat for at least two hours before exercising because elevated insulin levels may counteract the release of growth hormone.

The benefits of exercise

In an anti-ageing program, the goal of exercise is to increase flexibility, boost aerobic capacity and enhance strength. These three outcomes will result in muscle toning, loss of excess fat, increased muscle mass and optimisation of your muscle's use of oxygen and nutrients during rest and exercise — all of which will improve the appearance of your skin.

Along with weight (strength or resistance) training, some form of moderate aerobic exercise is equally beneficial. With heart-pumping aerobic exercise, your capillaries increase in size and number so that more oxygen and nutrients find their way to the skin and other tissues. Your skin will take on a healthy glow as a result.

Weight (strength) training:
- boosts metabolism (weight training can help 'reverse' the natural decline in your metabolism which begins around age thirty)
- promotes growth hormone secretion
- increases strength
- beefs up bone
- enhances energy
- improves moods
- perks up your posture.

In addition, heart-pumping cardio:
- increases your metabolic rate, which causes you to burn more kilojoules twenty-four hours a day
- improves cholesterol levels
- promotes growth hormone secretion
- boosts blood flow to your brain, increasing alertness
- enhances digestion
- reduces stress levels
- boosts your immune system resistance.

How much exercise is enough?

What kind of exercise and how much does it take to achieve these goals? The answer is: a variety of things, and less of them than you might think, but you must be dedicated. Swimming, weight training (with free weights or machines), running, bike riding, elliptical training machine (this is like a cross country skiing machine, which works your upper and lower body), walking, rollerblading, hiking, dancing, aerobics and even surfing are all great forms of exercise. Work towards a goal of exercising thirty minutes to one hour at least four to five days a week. Remember to always challenge yourself by adding variety to your workouts. This will help prevent you getting in an exercise rut, becoming bored and giving up. Pounding the pavements or the treadmill over the long term can eventually cause knee and lumbar spinal injuries, so try to vary your exercise as much as possible.

Don't forget to include weights, though, as even a slight increase in muscle mass boosts growth hormone and metabolism long-term (even while you sleep!) and that means extra kilojoules burned, even when you aren't working out. Most of your kilojoules are 'burned' by muscle tissue, so the more muscle you

A sample exercise session

Your exercise program should consist of about fifteen minutes of a slow and gentle warm-up, followed by twenty to forty minutes of fairly intense training, then a ten- to fifteen-minute cool-down period of moderate intensity. Alternate cardiovascular exercise (bike riding, elliptical machine or aerobics) with weight training (using free weights or machines). Try to alternate upper body strengthening exercises with back and lower body strengthening exercises. Finish off with some stretching to improve flexibility and relax your muscles. I would highly recommend a consultation with a personal trainer to make sure you're doing the exercises correctly and are adopting the right weight training program to suit your body shape.

Motivational music will really get you going, but switch off your mobile phone — this is also time to focus on you! Even if you think you have absolutely no spare time to exercise, I encourage you to make the time — the rewards for your body, beauty and mind will be enormous.

have, the faster your metabolism will be. One kilo of muscle burns up nine times the kilojoules of a kilo of fat!

Warning

Don't overdo it! Over-zealous and strenuous exercise has the opposite effect to what we want. When you exercise you use more oxygen and, in the process, you can create more free radicals; the long-term consequences may be faster ageing. Experimental work has shown that athletes display signs of higher free-radical induced cell damage than couch potatoes. Here's why: while exercising you take in many more times the oxygen than you would at rest, leading to an increased number of mitochondria in the cells of your muscles (the structures involved in your muscles' aerobic metabolism). The resulting mitochrondrial activity is thought to increase 'oxidation' and free radical production. Also, exercising in smoggy and polluted conditions can lead to an increased intake of ozone and nitrous oxide — nasty free radical generators. With the increased breathing during exercise, you are increasing the number of free radicals in your body. When the oxygen combines with the ozone or nitrous oxide, even greater numbers of free radicals are produced.

Excessive exercise doesn't only result in increased free radical activity; it also leads to elevated cortisol to DHEA ratios — an unfavourable con-

Fruitful workouts

Exercising in heat, sunlight, and pollution can increase oxidative stress. Researchers from the Appalachian State University in Boone, North Carolina, conducted a study to determine whether the potent antioxidants in blueberries could have an impact on reducing free radical load. The subjects were given a daily smoothie containing two-thirds of a cup of blueberries or a placebo. They were then exposed to high heat during exercise for two weeks and the results showed that the subjects who had the blueberry smoothie had eighty-three per cent less oxidative stress than the placebo drinkers! (Strawberries, blackberries, raspberries, prunes and raisins also have a high antioxidant content.) Lisa McAnulty, Assistant Professor of Food and Nutrition at the university, theorises that eating more antioxidants could guard against the damage caused by exercising in other hot environments, such as a Bikram yoga class.

dition, as we have seen. It seems the more strenuous the exercise, the more dramatic the increase in cortisol production. Remember, elevated cortisol levels reduce skin regeneration and can lead to accelerated wrinkling.

It's also interesting to note that moderate exercise will actually increase sex hormone production. But in a number of studies excessive exercise has been shown to decrease sex hormones. The key to exercise, like all things in life, is moderation and balance. Alternate exercise with yoga, Pilates and stretching and, of course, regular relaxation.

———————■———————

A key to ageing well is attitude. You are what you think. You can choose to be happy and enjoy life or be miserable. In his 2002 book *Ageing Well*, Dr George E. Valliant analysed three studies that followed 1400 people for sixty to eighty years. He found that those who lived the longest were the ones who had coped best with life's problems, even with traumatic events such as divorce and death of a loved one.

Anti-ageing begins at the cellular level, not on the surface of your skin, as many skincare companies would love you to believe. Short of surgery, there is no magical elixir for eternal youth. Growing old is a natural process which we will all undergo but you can determine how fast and how well you age by making a few simple choices: relax with yoga and meditation; experience the luxury of deep, restful sleep; and exercise in moderation for gorgeous, youthful skin. Because it's only when you are healthy internally — physically, mentally and emotionally — that your outer beauty will really shine.

6

Food and Lifestyle Sins

The Absolute Skin No-no's

Your skin doesn't lose its youthfulness overnight or on any particular birthday. It loses it in stages. In your late teens and twenties you could probably stay out all night, drink, smoke and wake up not looking a day older! Your skin would still look dewy and fresh. But somewhere in your thirties your skin stopped bouncing back after a big night out. As we age, cell turnover slows and the growth factors and hormones that made us bloom as adolescents begin to wane.

You experience moisture loss as sweat and oil gland production begins to decline. Meanwhile metabolism slows down within your cells, so the delivery of nutrients isn't quite so efficient and cellular wastes aren't eliminated as well. Gradually your skin becomes sluggish and loses its vital flow. Free-radical damage also accumulates from a variety of sources. Part of this is due to a decreased level of melanocytes (the cells that make melanin) and a corresponding lack of melanin secretion to protect your skin against sun-induced free-radical damage. Plus there's a natural decrease of GAGs (your moisture-holding molecules) in your dermal layer.

As you age, your skin produces less collagen, elastin and hylauronic acid — all crucial in keeping your face firm, smooth and youthful.

Fibroblasts (the mother cells of collagen and elastin) in your dermis also decrease each decade. Structural changes such as cross-linking take place in your collagen, which makes your skin less resilient. Your skin's immune system weakens, resulting in skin sensitivity, more vulnerability to injury and a longer healing time. What used to bounce back begins to sag. Static deep wrinkles may appear and our habitual expressions will, over time, leave their inevitable mark in the form of laugh and frown lines.

Over time the fat cells in your subcutaneous layer begin to decline, but they can accumulate in particular areas, resulting in bags under your eyes, enlarged ear lobes or a double chin! Elsewhere on the face, blood vessels and bones become increasingly visible as a result of an overall loss of fatty tissue. Also, when you have less fat under the skin, there is less padding to keep your skin plump and moist. Finally, you can lose that rosy glow, as there are fewer capillaries near the surface.

It's this combination of a thinning dermis, decreased collagen, diminished hydration levels, cross-linking and glycation that results in wrinkling and other signs of ageing. Generally you start to see the signs of ageing around age thirty to thirty-five but a multitude of factors can greatly speed up this process. The wrinkles on the surface of your skin are a reflection of changes in your dermal layer. Although the changes to your epidermis (outer layer) are quite subtle, the real action happens deep within. But this is also where you can have the most profound impact with diet and lifestyle too!

In this chapter we'll be looking at the food and lifestyle sins that can greatly speed up the ageing process and set you back in your pursuit of beautiful skin. Most of the food we unwittingly put in our mouths every day can create a combat zone for our skin. Blemishes, uneven skin tone, bags, dark circles and even premature ageing are a reflection of our diet and internal health. Each of the food sins discussed in this chapter has the potential to rob your skin of nutrients needed for vitality and tissue repair, to create inflammation and to accelerate free-radical damage and ultimately ageing.

While changing your diet can be one of the quickest ways to change your looks, it isn't the only key to maintaining naturally gorgeous skin for life. It's also crucial to avoid the key lifestyle enemies — cigarettes, excessive sun, stress, alcohol and caffeine. Ultimately the choices you make determine whether you shift into a high gear of accelerated ageing or not, and each of these lifestyle factors will set you back in your pursuit of beautiful skin.

Food sins
Skin enemy number one: sugar

A major sin against gorgeous skin is to consume any form of sugar. Sugar is listed by several names, sometimes incognito. Manufacturers try to disguise it by breaking up sugar counts, listing it as dextrose, high fructose corn syrup, sucrose, rice syrup, table sugar, honey, brown sugar, molasses and other forms of sweeteners to make the amount of sugar look less significant. Get sugar savvy and acquaint yourself with all the different forms of sugars.

The body breaks down all forms of sugar, natural and raw included, into the same molecules as white sugar, and they have the same number of kilojoules. And just in case you're reassuring yourself that your raw sugar is OK, you should know that one sugar is as bad as the other.

Track your sugar

You might want to keep a record of how many grams of sugar you consume in a day and you'll probably find that once you realise just how much sugar you're actually eating you'll automatically cut back. Add up the sugar grams listed on the labels of your food. Keep in mind that 28.4 grams is about two tablespoons. You can see it's so easy for sugar to creep into your diet — and it may shock you to really count how much sugar you're eating daily. Most commercial soft drinks contain about 1.2 teaspoons of sugar per 28 grams. Most cans contain 340 grams. That's a whopping 14.4 teaspoons of sugar, just in one can!

And sugar isn't easy to avoid. It sneaks into almost everything we eat — not just the obvious cakes, biscuits and soft drinks. In fact, it's hidden in virtually all packaged and processed foods. You name it — soups, cereals, sauces, tomato sauce, yoghurts and bread — it probably contains sugar.

Even if you don't add sugar to your coffee or indulge in cakes and biscuits, you'd be shocked at how much sugar you're actually eating every day. According to Elizabeth Somer, author of *The Origin Diet*, the average person in the United States eats between twenty-nine and forty teaspoons of refined sugar every day, or about 68 kilos per year![55] And in Australia the figures are not all that different.

Sugar may seem harmless enough, but it happens to be your worst skin enemy — for so many reasons. It robs cells of vital nutrients, generates free radicals, causes cross-linking of collagen, and results in youth-stealing spikes of insulin from high levels of blood sugar. (High blood sugar is like putting your foot flat to the floor on your ageing accelerator, and too much of it can blow your beauty big time.)

Insidious sweetness

According to Louise Gittleman, in her book *Get the Sugar Out*, foods containing 8 grams of sugar or more per serving should be eaten only on rare occasions. If you ate the following breakfast you would be getting well over 25 grams of sugar!

- A plate of fresh fruit
- A wholegrain wheat cereal that had sugar listed as the second ingredient and corn syrup as the sixth ingredient (sugar = 4 grams)
- A croissant — generally has sugar somewhere in the ingredient list
- Raspberry jam with sugar and corn syrup listed as the second and third ingredients
- Non-fat berry yoghurt — sugar being the second ingredient, modified corn starch the fourth (sugar = 19 grams)
- Low-fat milk
- A pat of butter.

Do you see how easy it is for sugar to slip unknowingly into your diet? Beware also of non-fat foods, as they're often packed with sugar to make them more appealing and all the more addictive.

Nutrient depletion

Processed sugar has been stripped of its nutritional value — fibre, vitamins and minerals — and in fact it robs your cells of much-needed nutrients. Important skin minerals such as chromium, manganese, zinc, cobalt and magnesium are lost in the process of refining sugar, and our bodies actually draw on their own mineral reserves just to digest and metabolise it. This results in an imbalance in certain important nutrients and also deficiencies in the B complex vitamins (vital for skin), all of which can lead to premature ageing.

According to Udo Erasmus, author and worldwide authority on essential fatty acids, 'sugar interferes with the transport of vitamin C … because both sugar and vitamin C use the same transport system'.[56] Remember that vitamin C is your prime beauty-boosting vitamin — vital for building collagen and elastin. So too much sugar will prevent vitamin C from performing its all-important task of helping to build up your skin's scaffolding, keeping it looking supple, radiant and line-free.

Avelin Kushi, author of *Diet for Natural Beauty* and wife of macrobiotics founder Michio Kushi, writes:

> simple sugars contribute to uneven colouring of the skin and are a leading cause of red blotches caused by overexpansion of blood capillaries near the surface, as well as freckles and large brown age spots. From a macrobiotic perspective these discolourations and pigmentation spots are caused by the 'expanding' effects of simple sugars. The depletion of calcium and other minerals caused by simple sugars also contributes to a loosening of the body's tissues and an overall puffiness and sagging of the skin.[57]

Cross-linking of collagen

When there is extra sugar floating around your bloodstream, its sticky sugar (glucose) molecules attach themselves to proteins and keep them from doing what they're supposed to do, setting the stage for cross-linking. How does this happen? Just think about when you spill sugar and try to wipe it up: it's sticky isn't it? The same thing happens in your body. It's that sticky attachment process that's called glycosylation, or glycation, and your collagen is the first to be affected. One of the fundamental processes of skin ageing, apart from free-radical damage and inflammation, is this process of glycation, because it actually causes cross-linking of collagen, which makes skin inflexible and prone to sagging, to discolourations such as age spots and to wrinkling. Cross-linking reactions are what cause an apple to turn brown and tough after you cut it up and are responsible for the hardening of a rubber mat or a garden hose left out in the sun. The same thing basically happens to your skin.

These new abnormal chemical structures are called advanced glycosylation end-products, or AGEs for short. You'll be hearing more about AGEs because a good deal of research has shown that they are destructive not only to the health and beauty of your skin but to every single organ in your body, your brain included.[58] When your collagen becomes glycosalated and AGEs form, the cross-linking destroys collagen's flexibility — so think sags, bags and wrinkles in your skin.[59] What's happening to your tissues from exposure to excessive glucose (sugar) is exactly what happens to meat when you brown it. In other words, you're slowly cooking yourself from the inside out — a sure-fire way for your skin to end up looking like a dried-out garden hose!

All is not lost, though. Exciting new research, detailed in Chapter 4, has shown that an anti-ageing supplement called Carnosine (not to be confused with L-carnitine) has the ability to bind to AGEs and inactivate them as well as block their actual formation. Carnosine rejuvenates connective tissue cells, and in doing so has a powerful effect on wrinkling. You can also help counter AGE formation by having small frequent meals with a low GI index and making sure they are also high in Omega-3 fatty acids and don't contain trans fats (see below).

Youth-stealing insulin spikes

You will especially want to give up sugar and refined carbohydrates if you have acne. In a recent study, researchers looked at 1200 natives of an island near Papua New Guinea and 115 hunter–gatherers in Paraguay and couldn't find a single pimple in the lot. What's their secret? 'A diet that consists almost exclusively of protein, fruits and vegies,' says Dr Loren Cordain, author of *The Paleo Diet*, professor of health and exercise science at Colorado State University and lead author of the study.[60] Absent from their meals were the simple carbohydrates, such as white bread, pasta, rice, potatoes and sweets, that are the basis of our modern diet. These carbohydrates send our insulin levels soaring, and researchers speculate that this sets off a series of reactions that leads to breakouts. The more refined the sugar, the faster the blood sugar level spike.

Eating refined carbohydrates and sugar also produces a surge of an insulin-like growth factor called IGF-1. This can lead to an excess of male hormones, which causes pores in the skin to secrete

Fruit juice fiction

Fructose, the natural sugar found in fruit, is different from cane sugar in that it has a very low GI of 25. But fruit *juices* are a different story.

If you think your daily glass of orange juice consumed on an empty stomach in the morning is healthy, think again! In the process of juicing fruit and vegetables, the fibre is removed and you're left with a high concentration of rapidly absorbable sugar. When this sugar hits your bloodstream it provokes a huge spike in your insulin levels. Go for whole fruit and vegetables, and if you do drink juices it's best to have them with a little food to blunt the insulin response.

If you can't give up your morning glass of juice, at least dilute half of it with water. This watered-down version won't taste so good the first few times you drink it, but your taste buds will get used to it. So much so that, later on, if you don't dilute your juice, it will probably taste too sweet.

Other sugar-related risks

Cutting out sugar has more than just beauty benefits. A study published in the Journal of the American Medical Association in January 2005 found that high levels of blood sugar are linked to cancer and diabetes, along with a higher mortality (death) risk.[61] A high blood sugar level was found to double the risk of pancreatic cancer. It's also interesting to note that tumour cells need glucose (sugar) for survival. So you'll be doing your health a huge favour by cutting out sugar. There's another major anti-ageing reason for wanting to avoid simple and refined carbohydrates: they can suppress growth hormone (HGH) release. Remember, you won't get far without human growth hormone (HGH). This key hormone (also known as somatotropin) is essential for maintaining proper brain function, energy levels, bone tissue and muscle mass, cell division, the repair of DNA within cells, and overall metabolism. Remember that refined carbohydrates and sugars boost insulin levels. When there's too much insulin in your blood, your body reacts by producing a chemical called somatostatin that suppresses insulin release. But it also suppresses HGH release.

sebum, a greasy substance that attracts acne-promoting bacteria. Also, IGF-1 causes skin cells known as keratinocytes to multiply, a process that is associated with acne.

Levels of insulin tend to rise with age too. This can be a cause of type 2 (adult onset) diabetes and a whole host of other inflammatory disorders. Remember, inflammation equals less-than-gorgeous skin. When insulin no longer moves sugar well (insulin resistance) both insulin and blood sugar levels rise. The excess blood sugar is then forced into your tissues, damaging them with AGEs.

Foods rich in complex carbohydrates — and low on the glycaemic index — don't trigger blood sugar spikes. These foods include beans, legumes, nuts and whole grains. (Nuts and seeds also contain an amino acid combination favourable to the production of growth hormone.)

While we're on the subject of HGH, an excess of dietary fat can also block the production and release of HGH, so it's best to limit fat intake to 20 to 30 per cent of your daily total kilojoules. Additionally, many longevity experts advocate reduced kilojoule intake and even occasional fasting as a good way to stimulate HGH production. The highest levels of growth hormone are released during sleep and during a fast that lasts for at least twenty-four hours.

! Note that fasting is not suitable for everyone, so always consult a
  health care professional before attempting a fast.)

The Gorgeous Skin program excludes every form of refined sugar —
from chocolate (except for the occasional piece of dark bittersweet
chocolate) to most jams to packaged breakfast cereals with their
hidden sugars. It does allow a little raw honey, stevia or xylitol for
sweetening.

Stevia is a kilojoule-free herb that is 150 to 400 times sweeter than
sugar and tends to have a slightly bitter aftertaste. Native to South
America, stevia has been used for centuries as a sweetener and flavour
enhancer and is sold in several forms in most health-food shops.

Xylitol is a safe, natural and healthy sugar substitute that has the
same sweetening power and taste as sugar but with no bitter aftertaste. It is a naturally occurring substance found in some plants,
fruits and vegetables. It is even produced by the human body as a
part of normal metabolism. Xylitol has a very low glycaemic index
of 7, so it won't increase blood sugar or insulin levels. You can use
it to satisfy your sweet tooth!

Artificial sweeteners — the bitter truth

Don't get lured into thinking that artificial sweeteners are any better
than sugar-based sweeteners. In fact, they pose a deadly threat to
your health and therefore your skin. Artificial sweeteners are also
referred to as non-nutritive or kilojoule-free sweeteners, and they are
intensely sweet synthetic substances, often used in place of other
sugars in food manufacturing and cooking because they are
kilojoule-free. But being kilojoule-free does not equate with weight
loss — or health, for that matter.

Axe the aspartame

Two hundred times sweeter than sugar, and without saccharin's bitter aftertaste, aspartame is cheered as the clear winner in the sugar substitute stakes by a diet-obsessed public. But it's actually a clear loser, for so many reasons. Known by various brand names, including Nutra-Sweet and Equal, aspartame is a chemical compound comprising phenylalanine, aspartic acid and methyl alcohol or methanol. When aspartame breaks down in the heat or when it's stored for too long, methanol (wood alcohol) is formed — not something you want to be eating if you're trying to reverse ageing! Aspartame is found in some four thousand products worldwide, including:

- soft drinks
- breath mints
- cereals
- sugar-free chewing gum
- cocoa mixes
- coffee beverages
- some pre-packaged desserts
- juice beverages
- laxatives
- multivitamins
- milk drinks/shake mixes
- pharmaceuticals and supplements
- tabletop sweeteners
- instant breakfasts
- yoghurts
- topping mixes
- instant teas and coffees.

Aspartame is believed to be by far the most dangerous food-additive on the market today. Symptoms attributed to aspartame include: severe headaches, nausea, vertigo, insomnia, loss of control of limbs, blurred vision, blindness, memory loss, slurred speech, mild to severe depression, hyperactivity, numbness, mood changes, loss of energy, ringing in the ears, loss or change of taste, and symptoms resembling a heart attack![62]

The major selling point of aspartame is as a diet aid — yet, ironically, research suggests that aspartame and other sugar substitutes make little difference in the battle of the bulge. Despite the widespread consumption of artificial sweeteners, the epidemic of obesity continues unabated. Studies have shown that the use of artificial sweet-eners actually causes people to eat more![63] Normally, when you eat enough carbohydrates, serotonin is released in the brain and you get that relaxed feeling after the meal. But when you combine aspartame with carbohydrates — for example, when you eat a sandwich with a Diet Coke — aspartame causes the brain to stop production of serotonin, meaning that you don't get that feeling of having had enough. You then eat more food, and often more containing aspartame, and the cycle continues.

Aspartame is officially not recommended for pregnant or lactating women, as its effects can be passed on to the developing foetus and the baby, even in very small doses. So if it's not suitable for growing babies, it shouldn't be recommended for anyone! If you see 'SUGAR FREE' on the label of a sweet, processed food, suspect the presence of aspartame … and read further.

Beauty-busting fats and oils

As we have seen, the types of fats and oils you eat can make the difference between having radiantly gorgeous, dewy skin and having sallow, dry, lacklustre skin. The 'bad' skin fats and oils will give you all or some of the following: greasy or large pores, acne, pimples and dry and flaky skin, dehydration or premature ageing — which will set you back big time in your pursuit of beautiful skin.

Just to recap, the 'bad' skin fats are:
- Trans fats which include hydrogenated and partially hydrogenated oils (e.g. margarine and vegetable shortening)
- oils used in deep or shallow frying
- polyunsaturated oils consumed in excess
- saturated fats
- cottonseed oil
- full-fat dairy products, including ice-cream.

Consuming large amounts of bad fats dramatically increases your body's free-radical load. The reason: when bombarded by free radicals, fat molecules split apart. The weak bond that holds together polyunsaturated fat molecules is especially sensitive and is readily broken down by heat, light and oxygen. So the more fat you eat, the more free radicals your body tends to generate. This is one major reason why heart disease and cancer, two conditions associated with cumulative free-radical damage, are most common in people who consume high-fat diets.

Trans fats: a trap

What makes trans fats so bad for your skin? First, let's take a look at what they are. Trans fats (also known as trans fatty acids) are polyunsaturated vegetable oils that have been chemically modified, via a process called hydrogenation, to make them solid at room temperature and to prolong shelf life. Trans fatty acids are also found in minor amounts (usually less than 2 per cent) in fats such as that from beef, pork and lamb. But the vast majority of trans fats are found in partially hydrogenated vegetable oils, which is basically a synthetic fat brimming with free radicals.

Trans fats are found in most processed foods, especially baked goods, where they are not labelled as trans fats. Instead, you'll see them listed as partially hydrogenated oil or just plain hydrogenated oil. Go into any supermarket and read the ingredient list on just about any package, even the so-called wholegrain breads and super-premium biscuits. Partially hydrogenated vegetable oils are sure to be in the top three or four ingredients. You'll also find trans fats in all sorts of other prepared foods, including: mayonnaise, salad dressings, donuts, chocolate bars, pretzels, processed cheese, potato chips, most brands of peanut butter, and of course in margarine.

All hydrogenated vegetable oils are free-radical bombs that

explode the moment you ingest them. Since high heat causes oils to oxidise even faster, all deep-fried foods are loaded with free radicals.

According to Dr Denham Harman (the originator of the free radical theory of ageing) and many other scientists, it is the oxidation of fats in the human body that's the primary cause of the cellular pathology associated with ageing. These artificial fats oxidise immediately upon exposure to air — the

Mischievous margarine

Margarine is major trans-fat trap. Because the fats in margarine are partially hydrogenated, manufactures can claim that it's 'polyunsaturated' and market it as healthy, but it isn't, by a long shot. Hydrogenation and partial hydrogenation produce dozens of nasty non-natural chemicals and a fiesta of free radicals. If that isn't bad enough, margarine is also a source of nickel and aluminium!

A little unsalted butter is always a safer bet than margarine. When in doubt always opt for the least processed or chemically altered alternative.

moment you unseal the can or bottle — and they continue to oxidise inside your system, setting up a chain reaction of molecular mayhem that can destroy cells and disrupt vital functions much faster than your body's natural capacity to defend itself from damage. Also, trans fatty acids do much of their damage by interfering with the body's handling of anti-inflammatory fats, specifically the Omega-3s.

Any food fried in polyunsaturated oil is cooked in trans fats. Whenever you deep-fry foods in corn, safflower, peanut or other common polyunsaturated oils, you're creating trans fats, and the foods you've cooked are much worse for you. So even if a product is cholesterol-free — which all vegetable oils are — it's still loaded with trans fats. Trans fats are a trap because companies advertise their biscuits and crackers as 'baked, not fried', or as having 'no saturated fat' or 'no cholesterol.' This implies they're low in fat, when in fact they're often full of trans fats. It doesn't matter if the product is cholesterol free; if it contains trans fat, it can age you and your skin.

Dr Barry Sears, author of *The Anti-ageing Zone*, calls trans fats the 'anti' essential fatty acids because of their destructive action in the body. The fats you eat make up the majority of your cell walls (membranes) and the problem with loading up on trans fats is that they end up being deposited in parts of your cell walls that should really be filled by your 'good' fats: the EFAs. So basically you're displacing your essential EFAs with terrible trans fats in your cell walls. When enough trans fats build up in your cell walls, they can become stiff and inflexible, causing a myriad of problems. Inflexible cell walls make it so much more difficult for nutrients to pass through and feed your cells, your skin cells included. Circulation can also become sluggish and this can ultimately lead to greasy pores, acne and dry, flaky skin.

Stiff cell walls also mean that cells can become less responsive to messages from your hormones and other important molecules. A by-product of this can be that your red blood cells become less responsive to insulin, and in doing so, in response to high levels of blood sugar, can make you pump out more inflammatory, ageing insulin than normal. Double bad news for skin.

Combine a diet high in refined sugar and carbohydrates plus trans fats — basically your average Western diet — and what do you get? A complete recipe for disaster as far as your skin is concerned.

Many fast foods are practically nothing but trans fats. A large order of chips at a fast-food restaurant could easily contain 7 grams of trans fats. And according to Elizabeth Somer, author of *The Origin Diet*, Americans are now eating 10 to 20 grams of trans fats every day. And if you eat enough potato chips, pretzels, biscuits, crackers or fried fast foods you would easily be averaging the 100 gram a day mark! Another reason to avoid trans fats is that in terms of general health, they have a nasty habit of raising levels of your bad fats and cholesterol. It's interesting to note that Denmark is one of the first countries to effectively ban all partially hydrogenated vegetable oils!

Fried foods

Avoid fried food like the plague. Heating oils to high temperatures produces many toxic substances, not just trans fats. When you cook unsaturated oils like corn, safflower or sunflower oil at high temperatures in the presence of oxygen (as in deep frying) this accelerates the production of lipid peroxides — major free-radical generators and age accelerators.

If you are having complexion problems such as pimples, open pores or acne, you will especially want to avoid any oil that has been heated. Quick stir-frying, with the addition of antioxidant rich garlic, is fairly safe, but slow cooking in high-temperature oil — that is, deep or shallow frying — is not.

Excessive polyunsaturated fats

Excessive polyunsaturated fats and oils can promote ageing. A study at the Irvine University in California examined the degree of wrinkling, crow's feet, frown lines and other indications of skin degeneration, such as damage to the collagen and elastin fibres, and the irregular pigmentation characteristic of older skin. The study found there was an undeniable link between marked clinical signs of ageing and a high intake of polyunsaturated fats in one's diet.[64]

Why? Polyunsaturated vegetable oils are highly unstable. This means that when cooked or left in a cabinet that gets hot or allows sunlight in, the oil can break down. It starts to oxidise or turn rancid much more quickly than other fats, generating huge amounts of age-accelerating free radicals that can damage our skin cells and manifest in increased wrinkles and even cancer. In fact all fats and oils produce free radicals when they oxidise (combine with oxygen) and break down. Natural fats such as butter, some meats and cold-pressed nut oils tend to oxidise much more slowly and produce far fewer free radicals than polyunsaturated fats.

Polyunsaturated oils occur naturally in whole grains and seeds, where they are accompanied by protective antioxidants, most notably vitamin E. However, when vegetable oils are processed, even the cold-pressed variety, they are usually robbed of their protective vitamin E content. The collagen fibres in skin are prime targets for free radicals, which cause them to bind together and become disorganised, resulting in lines and furrows. Vitamin E helps to minimise damage done by free radical chain reactions triggered by these fats.

Another problem is that in recent years Australians have increased the amount of polyunsaturated oils in their diet. We are eating more convenience, take-away, packaged and fried foods. A high intake of these polyunsaturated fats throws off the EFA balance, favouring the pro-inflammatory Omega-6s.

So, as a rule of thumb, as you increase the polyunsaturated oils in your diet, you should also be increasing your intake of vitamin E, vitamin C, beta-carotene and other protective phytonutrient antioxidants to neutralise these nasty free radicals and to naturally slow down the ageing of your skin.

Saturated fat

A mainstay in red meat, ice-cream and full-fat dairy, saturated fat can spark the production of free-radicals, which contributes to skin ageing. And according to one dermatologist, saturated fats inflame skin, inviting puffy pores and potentially angry pimples.[65] Another good reason to slow down on the saturates is that eating less saturated fat can help you maintain or increase your levels of youth hormones. As explained by the president of the American Anti-ageing Foundation, Dr Vincent Giampapa, 'we can encourage our bodies' production of youth hormones by getting no more than 10 per cent of our daily calories from saturated fat'.[66] In other words, if you con-

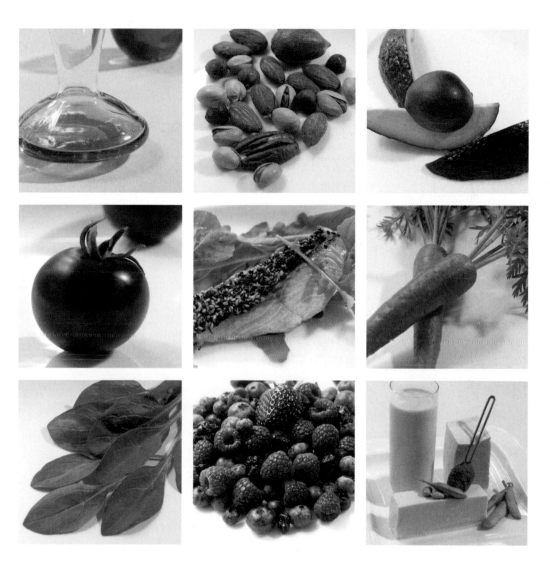

skin beauty boost

Give your skin a beauty boost with foods rich in vitamins, minerals, antioxidants, phytonutrients, and good protein and fats.

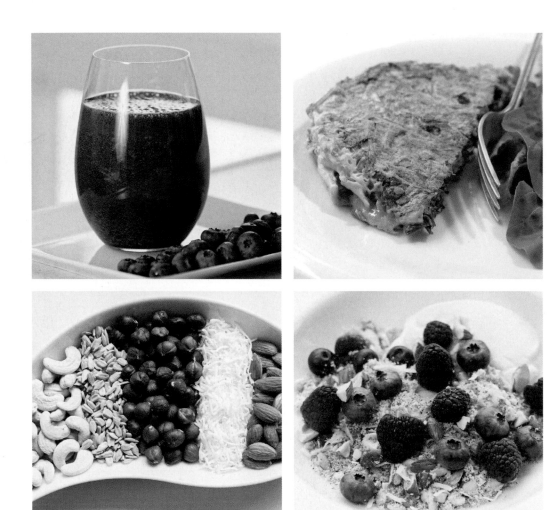

the perfect start

Start your day with the antioxidant-rich **Whey protein blueberry shake**, a delicious **Spinach frittata** full of protein and phytonutrients or the beneficial oils of the hearty **Cavewoman muesli**.

ingredients for cavewoman muesli shown bottom left

sume 7560 kilojoules in a day, no more than 756 of them (about 16–20 grams) should come from saturated fat. So steer clear of the saturates for supple, silky skin.

Reducing the amount of bad fats can have a profound impact on inflammatory skin conditions, too, such as psoriasis, eczema and dermatitis. Also, by replacing trans and saturated fats with good fats, you'll be decreasing your risk of developing skin cancer.

So how do you avoid unhealthy, ageing fats? Your best bet is to steer clear of all fast food — especially the fried kind. And when you're grocery shopping, check all the nutritional information labels for hydrogenated and partially hydrogenated oils.

Cottonseed oil

Cottonseed oil, found commonly in potato chips and other processed food, should be avoided at all costs as it contains toxic natural ingredients as well as huge amounts of pesticide residues. Pesticides are notorious free-radical generators.

Full-fat dairy products

Milk can also be a hidden source of saturated fat, depending on the type (whole, 2 per cent, 1 per cent, skim). The higher the fat percentage in milk, the greater the amount of saturated fat. Remember, what is true for milk is basically true for any dairy product (yoghurt, cheese, ice-cream, and so on). So, apart from natural yoghurt and kefir, steer clear of most dairy products.

A fat-free diet

A fat-free diet is a big-time beauty sin. Living on lettuce, fat-free yoghurt, bagels, diet soft drinks, non-fat salad dressings, low-fat or

The deceptive side of dairy

Dairy products have a relatively low glycaemic index compared with other foods such as bread. So you would expect that when you consume dairy products your insulin output would also be quite low. But recent research has shown that milk (both skim and whole milk) causes a strong insulin response, even though it has a low-glycaemic index.[67] In fact, the insulinaemic index of milk products hovers between 90 and 98, which actually isn't that different from the insulinaemic index of white bread! It seems that some milk component, along with the lactose (a sugar that naturally occurs in milk), stimulates the secretion of insulin.

There is one bright note, however. One of the studies showed that fermented products such as yoghurt had a lower insulin response than milk. The Gorgeous Skin program aims to control or reduce your levels of age-accelerating insulin, so that's why apart from fermented products such as natural yoghurt and kefir, dairy generally isn't recommend during the 30-day plan.

 TIP

Replace milk with organic soy, almond milk or rice milk. And good as full-fat ice-cream tastes, your skin will love you forever if you opt for fresh fruit and natural yoghurt instead.

non-fat biscuits and rice cakes for the sake of your weight will ravage your looks and ultimately cost you your beauty. Your skin needs 'good' fats to look lustrous, silky and supple. And a deficiency of EFAs can have a devastating effect on your skin and will eventually lead to an imbalance in your hormones, resulting in skin problems such as dryness, itching, eczema, scaling and thinning. This sort of diet lacks the beauty-enhancing EFA oils such as Omega-3 and Omega-6 (in moderation) that give you plump, luminous, smooth skin by aiding the absorption of your beautifying vitamins A, D, E and K, helping produce hormones and transporting oxygen throughout the body. Trading off your skin for weight loss may not show up straight away, but eventually your skin will look sallow and gaunt and will be prone to wrinkling, dark circles and thinning. Not a pretty picture.

Food sins summary: The absolute skin no-no's

SUGARS

- Dextrose
- Glucose
- High-fructose corn syrup
- Maltose
- Sucrose
- Table/raw/brown sugar

REFINED CARBOHYDRATES

- Bagels/Donuts
- Breakfast cereals
- Cakes/biscuits
- Pastries
- Sweets
- White bread
- White pasta
- White rice

HIGH-GI CARBOHYDRATES

- Baked/boiled potatoes
- Pretzels
- Rice cakes
- Tofu frozen dessert
- White bread
- White/instant rice

SOFT DRINKS

- All commercial soft drinks
- All diet soft drinks

ARTIFICIAL SWEETENERS

- Aspartame
- Sucralose

'BAD' SKIN FATS

- Cottonseed oil
- Excessive polyunsaturated fats
- Fried foods
- Full-fat dairy
- Margarine and shortening
- Saturated fats — processed meats
- Trans fats (hydrogenated and partially hydrogenated oils)

Lifestyle sins
Beauty Buster #1: cigarettes

If you can't manage to quit smoking cigarettes for health reasons, maybe vanity will motivate you. The long-term effects of smoking on your appearance might not yet be visible, but stop now and you'll be side-stepping the deeply grooved crow's feet, vertical furrows above the lips, broken capillaries, thinning skin and the trademark grey hue to the complexion that all smokers suffer.

Smokers develop their own particular brand of wrinkles, known as 'smoker's lines'. The pursing of the lips and squinting that accompany the inhaling and exhaling of toxic smoke etch permanent wrinkles on their faces, particularly around their mouths — not an appealing look. British doctor Douglas Model linked these distinctive characteristics to the effects of smoking, and in 1985 the diagnosis 'smoker's face' was even added to the medical lexicon.

The main reason that cigarette smoke is toxic to your skin is that four thousand beauty-busting chemical compounds are produced when tobacco burns! Also, the nicotine in cigarettes constricts blood vessels and deprives your cells of oxygen and nutrients, all of which can make your face look as ashen as the tip of a cigarette. Studies show that during smoking there's a thirty per cent decrease in oxygen supply to your skin. When your skin is deprived of oxygen and nutrients, each and every skin cell is starved of the factors that it desperately needs to repair itself and to look as good as possible.

Cigarette smoke is also hazardous to the healthy turnover of your skin cells. Normally, skin enzymes known as matrix metalloproteinases (MMPs) continually break down old collagen — connective tissue fibres — to make way for new collagen. Skin deprived of collagen loses its elasticity, so a smoker's skin will eventually look shrivelled, dull, blotchy and of course heavily wrinkled.

In a recent test-tube study, researchers at Nagoya City University

Medical School in Japan exposed skin cells to a salt-water solution infused with cigarette smoke. The skin cells in the smoky fluid acted abnormally, churning out more collagen-destroying MMP enzymes than usual, while the formation of new collagen dropped by a whopping forty per cent! The famous 'twin studies' have also shown that, after several decades, smokers' skin becomes about forty per cent thinner than it should be. The thinner the skin, the weaker the connective tissue and the more saggy and wrinkled it appears. Obviously, smoking is a total no-win situation for skin.

A substance in cigarette smoke called benzopyrene also makes the skin age rapidly. Benzopyrene uses up your body's supply of vitamin C at great speed, making it unavailable for the support of healthy collagen and causing skin to wrinkle far earlier than it should. Remember that vitamin C is the number one collagen-building nutrient. Each and every cigarette robs your body of an estimated 25 milligrams of vitamin C — far too many withdrawals from the beauty bankbook!

Along with all the other noxious, beauty-destroying chemicals it supplies, smoking also increases blood levels of free radicals, which can damage collagen and elastin, the proteins that hold the skin together. Every puff generates an astounding 100 trillion radicals. If your body is not primed with huge amounts of antioxidants, smoking-induced free-radical damage causes small puckers or gathers to develop. These puckers crimp the skin, along with the collagen and elastin that lies beneath it, and result in what we observe as a wrinkle.

Yet another problem is the carbon monoxide in the air from the residue of smoking — second-hand smoke and its aftermath. It binds together with the red blood cells' haemoglobin, tying up its oxygen-carrying capacity for about twelve hours. This can lead to oxygen starvation in the skin's cells and make radiantly beautiful skin a sheer impossibility!

According to Paula Begoun, author of *The Beauty Bible*, 'cigarettes are probably even more insidious than sun exposure when it comes to healthy skin'.[68] Not only does smoking literally suffocate the skin, reducing oxygen in the blood by replacing it with carbon monoxide and causing serious free-radical damage, it also creates necrotic (dead) skin tissue that cannot be repaired. Even more unattractive is the breakdown of the elastic fibres of the skin (elastosis) which gives rise to yellow, irregularly thickened skin.[69]

While all of these factors can make skin look prematurely wrinkled and aged, smoking is also unattractive for many other reasons, including the permeating smell of smoke in hair and on clothing, smoker's breath, and the tell-tale yellow stains on hands, nails and teeth. Smoking isn't pretty and, as the label on the pack states, it really can kill you.

Another beautiful reason to quit smoking

In October 2002, scientists at the Scripps Research Institute in La Jolla California announced that smoking accelerates the glycation process. They found that a by-product of nicotine causes an accelerated 'cooking' of protein and the formation of health and skin destroying AGEs.[70] This discovery should give smokers concerned with both beauty and health even more incentive to kick the habit!

Even if you don't smoke, don't be quick to assume you are escaping the devastating effects of cigarettes. Passive smoking also has a big impact on skin. Eighty-eight per cent of non-smokers show signs in their blood of cotinine, a chemical that comes only from breathing in cigarette smoke.[71] And just by being in a room with smokers, you can take in considerable quantities of benzopyrene, tar, carbon monoxide and other irritating substances … so give smoking the boot!

Beauty Buster #2: excessive sun

The sun can be incredibly seductive and we really do seem to feel sexier and more vital when we have sun-kissed skin. We also need sunshine to regulate our sleep–wake cycles and enhance our feel-good factor. There is a scientific reason for all of this. Sunlight activates a gene called pom-C, which in turn helps create melanin and enhances sex drive; the endorphins or 'happiness hormones'; and leptin, which helps you burn fat.

The production of melanin in the skin creates a powerful protective antioxidant system. It actually protects the nuclear structures in your skin cells from damaging UV rays. When UV rays assault your skin, melanin migrates into your individual skin cells to form a physical umbrella over its nucleus that protects it from sun damage. It takes about three days to induce significant melanin in your skin. During this process your skin darkens with repeated exposure to UV light — a reaction that produces a suntan. Sun tanning in effect puts your skin's melanin production into overdrive to protect your skin from burning. Melanin is also a potent neutraliser of skin-ageing free radicals. In addition, the skin's natural defences against oxygen radicals include other antioxidants such as vitamin E and beta-carotene, and the copper-containing protein superoxide dismutase, all of which detoxify oxygen radicals and reduce skin damage.

And we absolutely need sunshine to stay healthy and for the production of vitamin D — the sunshine vitamin — critical for developing bones and for absorbing and using calcium, which in turn helps prevent osteoporosis and many other forms of cancer (including breast and colon cancer and even possibly melanoma!). Most of the body's vitamin D supply — about 75 per cent of it — is generated by the skin's exposure to UV rays.

But too much sun is right up there with cigarettes as one of the worst destroyers and agers of skin that we're likely to encounter. If you're not convinced, compare your unexposed skin (such as the skin on the inside of your arms, buttocks or breasts) with the skin on your face or arms. Quite probably, it's still soft and baby-smooth, because it has rarely seen the light of day.

According to the CSIRO, the ozone layer, which protects the earth from ultraviolet radiation, has decreased over Australia by close to 10 per cent during the last twenty years. And with every one per cent loss of ozone, there's a corresponding two per cent increase in UV rays reaching the ground. It might not sound like much, but it can certainly damage your skin and age you prematurely.

The real problem is that not only does too much sunshine accelerate the visible ageing of your skin, it also destroys the physical integrity of your skin. (There are two kinds of UV rays: UVA rays accelerate the signs of premature ageing by reducing the skin's firmness and elasticity, while UVB rays are responsible for burning.) The skin's first defence against UV rays is the barrier of the skin itself. A second barrier is provided by your body's naturally occurring antioxidants and repair mechanisms. And the last line of defence is your skin's immune system, which neutralises or destroys potentially foreign and dangerous substances like free radicals. All of these barriers, especially the immune system, are under attack from increased exposure to UV radiation.

The sun first attacks the epidermis (your outermost layer of skin). Over time, it also damages the upper layers of the dermis, leaving it thinner, less resilient and more susceptible to wrinkling. Collagen and elastin fibres that form the dermis also become disorganised and begin to break down, conspiring with gravity to cause gradual drooping and sagging.

If photo-ageing continues, collagen production in the dermis falls off at a rate of about one per cent per year. Changes occur in skin cells too. Keratinocytes are damaged; melanocytes (the cells that produce the pigment melanin) are gradually killed off; and your outside skin layer, the epidermis, thickens. Other visual legacies of sun damage include age spots, spider veins, dilated capillaries, crow's feet, sagging jowls, leathery skin, dull skin and an uneven skin tone.

When the sun's UV rays penetrate the top layers of your skin, free radicals are produced, which in turn oxidise lipids (fat substances) in your cell membranes, creating destructive chain reactions. These free radicals can stimulate the release of inflammatory agents as well as the production of enzymes such as collagenase. Collagenase is the enzyme that destroys collagen! So too much sun is a no-win situation for your skin.

UV rays are not only insidious generators of free radials; they also deplete antioxidants. People with skin cancer have suboptimal levels of vitamin C, which is a chief antioxidant in skin. Studies have shown that exposure to UV radiation (or 'sunburn' radiation — the equivalent of forty-five minutes of noonday sun) or smog depletes 80 per cent of your skin's vitamin C stores. So people who live in sunny, smoggy places like Sydney or LA get a double whammy!

When it comes to withstanding the effects of the sun, people with darker complexions usually have the least sun damage because the pigment melanin in their epidermal layer absorbs the UV light, shielding their skin from damage. The amount of melanin our skin produces determines our level of natural protection. Dark-skinned people have naturally higher levels of melanin in their skin, but in fair-skinned people extra melanin often promotes the development of freckles and sun spots. So the most vulnerable to skin damage are women with fair skin and light hair and eyes, as well as women who have grown up living at high altitudes, where UV rays are most intense, and of course those living under the harsh Australian sun.

The melanoma mystery

Australia has the highest incidence of skin cancer in the world. In fact, one in two Australians will develop some form of skin cancer

Tanning bed trauma

The rays from a tanning salon are certainly not safer than lying in the sun, and it's not possible to avoid UV damage by using tanning booths or sunlamps, as the rays from those sources are equally harmful. A Johns Hopkins University study found that skin cells of tanning-bed enthusiasts undergo molecular changes that raise the risk of skin cancer. Cells in exposed skin showed a significant increase in the most common kind of DNA damage, caused by sunlight: cyclobutane pyrimidine dimer (CPD), which if not repaired by the body, causes skin-cell mutations that can lead to cancer.[73] So don't get cheated into believing tanning beds are a safe alternative.

during their lifetime and more than 382,000 Australians are diagnosed with skin cancer each year. Of those, 8500 are diagnosed with the deadly form of melanoma skin cancer, with 1300 dying each year. Basal cell and squamous cell cancers are closely linked to lifetime sun exposure, yet they rarely kill. Melanomas are the problem skin cancer and can certainly be deadly, but it seems that our modern diet rather than sunlight is the guilty party. Worldwide, the greatest rise in melanoma has been experienced in countries where chemical sunscreens have been heavily promoted. Although the medical establishment still strongly supports the use of sunscreens there is a growing consensus among progressive researchers that the use of sunscreens does NOT prevent skin cancer and, in fact, may actually promote skin cancers as well as colon and breast cancer.[72] It's interesting to note that the rise in melanoma has been exceptionally high in Queensland where the medical establishment has vigorously promoted the use of sunscreens. Queensland now has more incidences of melanoma per capita than any other place on Earth.

Research published in 2001 in the United States revealed that excessive amounts of Omega-6 oils such as corn oil, safflower, sunflower, sesame, soya and canola oil — and not the sun — may actually be triggering skin cancers![78] On the other hand Omega-3 fats like flaxseed and other fish oils may actually help prevent melanoma. An Australian study done ten years ago showed a 40 per cent reduction in melanoma for people who eat fish regularly![79] Other studies have

Screen your sunscreen

Sunscreens are designed to protect against sunburn (UVB rays) and generally provide little protection against UVA rays. They come in two forms: chemical and physical. Chemical sunscreens prevent sunburn by absorbing the ultraviolet (UVB) rays. Chemicals such as avobenzone, benzophenone (or its derivatives oxybenzone and benzophenone-3), ethylhexyl p-methoxcinnimate, 2-ethylhexyl salicylate, homosalate and octyl methoxycinnamate are used as the active ingredients. (It's believed that they may increase the risk of cancers of the breast, ovaries, prostate and colon.)

Physical sunscreens contain inert minerals such as titanium dioxide, zinc oxide or talc and work by reflecting the ultraviolet (UVA and UVB) and visible rays away from the skin.

Progressive Canadian researcher and chemist Hans Larsen believes that chemical sunscreens may actually help promote skin cancer, by virtue of their free-radical generating properties. In an article published in the International Journal of Alternative and Complementary Medicine, Larsen noted that 'Benzophenone is one of the most powerful free radical generators known to man.'[74]

Doctors Cedric and Frank Garland of the University of California also believe that the increased use of chemical sunscreens is the primary cause of the current skin cancer epidemic seen in Australia and the Western world. According to the Garlands, the greatest rise in melanoma has actually occurred in countries where chemical sunscreens have been heavily promoted. They contend that physical sunscreens are much safer for the skin.[75]

The Norwegian Radiation Protection Authority conducted a study and found that a weak dose of OMC (octyl methoxycinnamate), a chemical used in 90 per cent of sunscreens, killed half the mouse cells it touched.[76] Shining a lamp on the OMC-pregnated cells to simulate sunshine made the chemical even deadlier. In the tests, the concentration of OMC was only five parts per million, a much lower concentration than that used in sunscreens! More than 90 per cent of the cells survived in the solution without OMC.

Even more alarming is research conducted at the Institute of Pharmacology and Toxicology, University of Zurich, Switzerland, which found that many widely used sunscreen chemicals can mimic the effects of oestrogen and trigger developmental abnormalities in rats! One of the most common sunscreens, 4-MBC, when mixed with olive oil and applied to rat skin, caused a doubling of the rate of uterine growth well before puberty.[77] And we're still being told to slather these chemical sunscreens not only on ourselves but also on young children!

So do read sunscreen labels carefully, and for the sake of your skin and your general health opt for a physical sun block containing titanium dioxide and zinc oxide. (See Resources, page 308, for details on non-chemical sunscreens.)

shown that people who eat the most fruits and vegetables have the lowest incidence of skin cancer and other cancers as well. So it seems that our modern diet is more to blame than the sun. This would explain why one recent case-controlled study of 966 patients found that lifetime sun exposure appeared to indicate a lower risk of malignant melanoma![80] And melanoma seems be more prevalent among city dwellers than among people who work out of doors. So make sure you eat lots of deep-sea fish, fresh fruit and vegetables and cut back on all refined Omega-6 oils including margarine.

Tips for safe sunning

If you do go out in the sun, wear a good non-chemical sunscreen. *never, ever* allow your skin to *burn*! The inflammation you see when you burn destroys the collagen and elastin network of fibres in your skin permanently, which leaves a legacy of thin, wrinkled skin ... much less glamorous in the long run than pale skin!

Avoid the sun altogether when UV radiation is strongest: between 10 a.m. and 4 p.m. (3 p.m. in winter). When you must be outdoors for a long while, use a broad-spectrum, non-chemical sunscreen with a rating of at least SPF 15 or, if possible, SPF 30. Remember that sunlight reflects strongly off sand, concrete and snow! Keep yourself covered. Put on a wide-brimmed hat (at least 10 centimetres in width) and sunglasses with full-spectrum, UV-filtering lenses. Wear long sleeves and long pants in the sun. And lastly, make sure to supplement your diet with additional vitamins and minerals, particularly C, D, E, mixed carotenoids including beta-carotene and selenium. These fight free-radical oxidation and can boost the immune system and help to protect against not only UV damage but also cancers and cataracts.

For a radiantly beautiful complexion, limit sun exposure to fifteen minutes, three times a week (mornings and late afternoons only).

Beauty Buster #3: stress

In today's world it's virtually impossible to live stress-free. Stress is ever-present in our lives: at work, in our relationships, driving through rush-hour traffic, through noise pollution, information overload, and fast-paced technological change. From the moment we get up in the morning, we hit the ground running, reading as we talk as we text message as we eat as we drive as we phone as we e-mail! We constantly juggle work commitments, family and our social life.

Most of us have come to accept the occurrence of stressful situations on a regular basis, day after day. And while we may think that we crave a leisurely life, the truth is that most of us are so culturally programmed to overcommit that even those of us who don't have an office to go to rarely feel completely unemployed! Women's lives in particular are so crammed full of commitments that many of us are running on empty. It's actually this long-term chronic stress that over-stimulates our hormonal and nervous systems, and which accelerates ageing of our bodies ... our skin included.

It's true that no two people respond to the same situation in the same way, and what one person may find stressful is not necessarily stressful for another. Stress in itself isn't such a negative thing; it gives us the drive to get out and accomplish things. It is our *response* to stress that can be destructive. So it isn't actually the stress that harms us directly; it's the accompanying distress that is so detrimental. Distress happens when we experience prolonged emotional stress and don't (or aren't able to) deal with it in a positive manner.

Our bodies react to stress in three phases:
- alarm
- resistance
- exhaustion.

The alarm phase is our 'fight or flight' response. The body releases a number of stress hormones, including one called cortisol, as it prepares to do battle. However, as modern-day stressors typically aren't physical things that we can fight or run away from, the alarm stage is prolonged, leading us into the next phases: resistance and then exhaustion. It's during this exhaustion phase that our body becomes 'distressed', which can result in everything from fatigue to accelerated ageing.

Normally our adrenal glands release just small amounts of cortisol in response to stress, thereby making it manageable. But excessive, unrelenting stress causes an overproduction of cortisol. Cortisol is often referred to as the 'pro-ageing hormone' because when it's secreted in high amounts over extended periods the inflammation process is stepped up, and in turn this can lead to a depressed immune function, a decrease in muscle mass, an increase in age-accelerating insulin and fat storage, plus thinning of the skin. Excess cortisol accelerates all forms of ageing and can be a major beauty buster.

A major key to maintaining a gorgeous, glowing complexion is to reduce the stress response and thereby bring down cortisol levels. (Strategies to help lower your cortisol levels are discussed at length in the next chapter.) Reducing stress levels also reduces levels of free radicals in your body — an important anti-ageing strategy. Learning to change how you react to situations, practising relaxation and meditation techniques and committing to a more positive, open attitude towards life can help keep you feeling years younger and provide a big boost for beautiful skin.

Long term, there are other ways in which relentless stress can greatly contribute to the ageing process. When stress activates your body's metabolic processes it causes you to use more oxygen, so you have a greater amount of oxidative stress, which means many more destructive free radicals. In turn this places a greater antioxidant demand on your nutritional defence system.

If we don't have a nutrient-rich diet, we generally don't get enough protective antioxidant nutrients and our body will be so much more susceptible to the harmful effects of free radicals. In other words, psychological stress combined with a poor diet can cause harmful free radicals to go unchecked and proliferate which can exacerbate their effects and in turn will affect our skin.

Chronic stress can also deplete your much-needed stores of beauty nutrients. Researchers at the United States Department of Agriculture measured blood mineral levels in people during a five-day period of severe psychological stress. Results showed that despite adequate dietary intake, blood levels of several minerals dropped as much as 33 per cent.

The key nutrients lost to stress are vitamin C — collagen booster extraordinaire — the B vitamins and magnesium. All are required for skin to look its radiant best. During chronic mental or physical stress, magnesium is released from your cells, from where it enters your bloodstream and is then excreted in your urine. The more stressed we are, the more magnesium we lose.

New research has found that this chronic stress affects the major biological factors involved with ageing at a cellular level: telomere length, telomere activity and oxidative stress.[81] Telomeres are the caps at the ends of your chromosomes that consist of DNA and protein. These telomeres naturally shorten with age but we have an enzyme in our body called telomerase, which protects and replenishes telomeres and in turn increases a cell's lifespan. The research found that oxidative stress, caused by excess free radical activity, damages the DNA and actually speeds up telomere shortening.

The study conducted by scientists at the University of California, San Francisco (UCSF) found that when telomere length was analysed, the people who perceived the greatest stress had the equivalent of ten years of additional ageing compared with participants who perceived the lowest stress levels. Decreased telomerase activity and increased oxidative stress were also significantly higher in the group who reported the most stress. Dr Elizabeth Blackburn, author, and Morris Herzstein, Professor of Biology and Physiology at

UCSF's Department of Biochemistry and Biophysics, commented: 'The results were striking. This is the first evidence that chronic psychological stress — and how a person perceives stress — may dampen down telomerase and have a significant impact on the length of telomeres, suggesting that stress may modulate the rate of cellular ageing.' As you can see, along with eating well, it's just as critical to manage your stress well. More on this and other stress-busting strategies in the next chapter.

Beauty Buster #4: alcohol

Most of you will be happy to know that there isn't any research to show that the moderate consumption of wine has a negative effect on health. In fact, studies have indicated that drinking a glass of wine — particularly red wine — each day may reduce the risk of cardiovascular disease because of the phenolic substances (such as the flavonoids and resveratrol) found in grapes.[82] The flavonoids found in wine (again, particularly red wine) also help scavenge toxins and free radicals. After testing hundreds of foods, scientists at the University of Illinois at Chicago found resveratrol (in red wine, red and white grapes and in 72 other plant species) to be one of the most potent cancer-preventing agents. Resveratrol has also been shown to slow down blood platelet aggregation (clumping) and the oxidation of LDL ('bad') cholesterol.

The antioxidants, particularly those in red wine, help maintain the elasticity of your arteries by reducing plaque build-up. Flexible arteries can dilate (expand) easily, ensuring good circulation to your skin. In fact, just one glass of wine promotes immediate vasodilation, bringing a rosy (but temporary) flush to your cheeks.

! Rosacea sufferers take note: alcohol causes the skin to flush, a sign that your capillaries are dilating. Normally, those thread-like vessels will shrink again, but if you suffer from rosacea, a skin condition that shows up as a persistent swath of redness on the face, you'll only aggravate the condition.

While it's true that the occasional glass of a good red wine may relax you and could improve your digestion and long-term health, drinking in excess is definitely not beneficial to your skin. Too much alcohol shows in a sallow complexion, puffy face and red eyes. Why? For one thing, alcohol is a diuretic; it dehydrates the body and can sap it of B vitamins. The all important B vitamins help keep nails hard, hair thick and skin clear and luminous. A deficiency of the B vitamins can also result in dry, thin skin.

Alcohol can also cause blood vessels to dilate, creating puffiness around the eyelids and a generally swollen appearance. Because of its diuretic effects, it increases leakage of blood vessels and capillaries, especially under the eyes, also leading to puffiness and redness of the lower eyelids. Another unattractive effect of alcohol is a lowered resting muscle tone, which can make the face look drawn.

Each gram of hard alcohol contains 30 kilojoules — more than any other type of food except fat — and the kilojoules it gives you are empty nutrition, as they convey no vitamins, minerals or essential nutrients to the cells of your body. This equates to 'minus' beauty points.

Excessive alcohol can also bring about sludging of the capillaries. So instead of the millions of red blood cells circulating freely, they tend to clump together and clog tiny blood vessels, interfering with circulation so that the cells don't get enough oxygen. As a result of this oxygen deprivation, cellular deterioration occurs and small haemorrhages take place. This 'sludging' phenomenon interferes with skin metabolism and with other cells elsewhere in the body. The tiny ruptures that take place in small blood vessels are a major factor behind the appearance of broken capillaries on the face.

If you do drink alcohol other than red wine during the program, make sure you take extra antioxidants and B vitamins and fend off dehydration by drinking a large glass of water for each alcoholic beverage you imbibe. And always make sure you eat when you drink alcohol.

Beauty Buster #5: caffeine

Caffeine is also a diuretic, so it saps your body and skin of moisture. Another problem with caffeine is that it activates your adrenal glands, raising your levels of stress hormones — especially the hormone cortisol (your 'pro-ageing' hormone that can lead to inflammation and, in the long term, to premature ageing).

Don't even think about decaf

Just in case you think about switching to decaf, think again. In the process of actually 'decaffeinating' the coffee, chemicals such as trichlorethylene or methylene chloride are used. These chemicals are major health and beauty busters.

I know personally how hard it is to kick the coffee habit, so if you can't forgo your caffeine entirely, try to reduce it to one cup per day, and down a glass of water with each cup of coffee to make up for its dehy-drating effects. Better yet, every second day trade your usual cup of coffee for antioxidant-rich green tea, herbal tea, or hot water with a squeeze of lemon juice. The different form of caffeine in green tea will give you a softer lift.

Green Tea is anti-inflammatory, meaning that it calms sensitive skin, and it's also rich in antioxidants. Studies have shown that it's also great for preventing and possibly even reversing sun damage! For radiantly beautiful skin, add teas and fresh juices to your daily beverage allotment, and limit yourself to just one cup of java.

Beauty Buster #6: sleep position

The position in which you routinely sleep has a significant effect on facial wrinkling — a fact that was discovered during sleep studies conducted in the early 1980s and confirmed recently in new research. If you typically sleep on your stomach (or even on your side) with your face pressed against your pillow — watch out! You could be adding bags, sags and years to your age. Medical research found that if you sleep eight hours or more with your face pressed against a pillow or the bed, creases will develop in your skin. These wrinkles tend to form across the forehead, down the side of the nose, as a horizontal line under the eyes, or as a long vertical line down the cheek. However, these lines are less likely to develop or become permanent if you routinely sleep on your back.

Beauty Buster #7: yo-yo dieting

Along with frying yourself in direct sunlight at noon, one of the other sure ways to get wrinkles fast is to put on lots of weight and then lose it quickly. Regardless of the cause, extreme weight gain or loss will have a huge impact on your skin. Weight gain stretches your skin. Once you drop the extra kilos, the skin remains loose rather than reverting to its original state. A major cause of this, other than just weight loss, is your age (this wouldn't have happened in your twenties or early thirties) and the years of earlier sun damage. Most women and men in their forties quickly and definitely start seeing increasing amounts of wrinkles and skin discolorations and a loss of firmness. Also keep in mind that gaining and losing weight in cycles may have other negative effects, not only on your skin but on your overall health as well.

7

Detoxification

Purifying Your Body and Skin

What do Liv Tyler, Christy Turlington, Demi Moore, Christy Brinkley, Madonna, Barbra Streisand, Uma Thurman and Ben Affleck have in common? They all enjoy the benefits of regular juice fasts and detox diets. And they all have gorgeous, glowing skin!

Devotees of detoxing claim they have more energy, improved sleep, greater mental clarity and clearer, more radiant skin. A short juice fast or detox is like giving your body an internal spring clean at the deep cellular level. By boosting your body's natural cleansing process and giving your digestive system (including your liver) a well-deserved rest, your body can focus on clearing out the stored toxins that have accumulated over the years.

To live a life of health and vitality, make the most of your good looks, and prolong your youth potential, one of the best things you can do is rid your body of toxic wastes through a short cleanse or detox. The detoxification program outlined in this chapter is designed to trigger a gentle yet effective detoxification and to kick-start your 30-day gorgeous skin program.

Detox – internal housekeeping

For a lot of people, the word detox conjures up images of struggles with alcohol and drugs, but detoxification is a natural process. In fact, internal detoxification is one of your body's most basic automatic functions. Just as your heart beats non-stop and your lungs breathe continuously, your metabolic processes constantly get rid of accumulated toxic matter that has built up in your cells, tissues and organs. You eliminate or neutralise toxins through your liver, kidneys, colon, lungs, lymph and skin every day. For example, when you drink a cup of coffee, your liver transforms the caffeine to a more harmless substance that can be eliminated in your urine.

A great detox program boosts your natural cleansing systems and encourages your body to rid itself of chemicals and toxic by-products that accumulate in your cells and tissues over the years. The consequences of poor eating habits, pollution, environmental chemicals, hormones and the usual suspects — cigarettes, drugs, alcohol and caffeine — need to be flushed from your system on a regular basis for your skin to look its best.

A detoxification program assists your body's natural cleaning process by:

- resting your organs (particularly your hard-worked digestive system)
- stimulating your liver to drive toxins from the body
- promoting elimination through your intestines, kidneys and skin
- improving circulation of your blood
- refuelling your body with healthy nutrients.

Beauty benefits

As your body responds to the three-day detox program you will notice the following beauty benefits.

- Your face will look rested, rejuvenated and revitalised.
- Your skin's natural glow will return as capillary circulation and lymphatic draining improve.
- Skin blemishes, blotches and spots will diminish or disappear.

- The whites of your eyes will become whiter.
- Dark under-eye circles will fade or disappear.
- Your skin texture will become smoother and softer.
- Fine lines will be less noticeable.

Other benefits of detoxing

What else do you get from a detoxification program? Giving your body the chance to clear out the rubbish it has been carrying will encourage weight loss (if you are overweight) and will help you to shed cellulite, improve overall muscle tone and increase your sense of vitality and wellbeing. It will cleanse your digestive system, restore a good acid–alkaline balance to your body and stimulate the proper functioning of your organs and tissues. A detox also encourages you to look at your diet and lifestyle, and to make positive long-term changes. In short, detoxification effects a transformation that leaves you feeling great and sparkling with vitality.

Why detox?

Detoxing isn't new. Fasting — a form of detoxification — is one of the oldest therapeutic practices in medicine. Hippocrates, the ancient Greek known as the 'Father of Western medicine', recommended fasting as a means of improving health. Ayurvedic medicine, a traditional healing system from India developed over thousands of years, also uses detoxification to prevent disease and treat many chronic conditions, including skin problems.

A toxin is any substance that irritates or causes harmful effects in your body. One cause of toxicity is the absorption of environmental toxins. We live in a toxic jungle where metabolic wastes and toxins work their way into our bodies faster than they can be eliminated. The United States chemical industry alone produces and releases about 400 kilos of chemicals per American per year, which end up in that country's water, its food chain, its atmosphere and ultimately the bodies of its population. American agriculture uses nearly 4.5 kilograms of pesticides per person on the food supply each year! In Australia we're not that far behind. Many of these dangerous chemicals, called volatile organic compounds (VOCs), are fat-soluble and concentrate in fat in your body and brain. These chemicals can interfere with your normal metabolic processes and cause symptoms such as 'brain fog' (inability to think clearly, poor memory, difficulty concentrating), fatigue, and malaise along with many others.

Toxicity can also be caused by the food we eat. Sugar, 'bad' fats, refined foods, alcohol, caffeine, second-hand smoke, pesticides, additives, preservatives, a nutrient-poor diet, cosmetics and even skin-care products contain toxins that can eventually build up in your body and prevent your skin from looking as good as it could.

A highly processed diet, a severely unbalanced diet, or simply too much food can also overburden your elimination and digestive systems. Some people are unable to digest food properly due to years of overeating and diets that are high in fat and processed foods, and low in fibre (the average Western diet)! Instead of being digested properly or eliminated from your colon, food can putrefy inside your digestive tract and produce toxic by-products! Not a pleasant thought, but it's very real! This is referred to as toxic colon syndrome or intestinal toxaemia.

Your digestive system isn't the only system affected. A diet high in 'bad' fats, alcohol, caffeine, sugar or the use of medications can also contribute to the burden on your liver — one of your key detoxification organs. Hormones and antibiotics fed to the animals that we eat, preservatives, dyes used in food processing, heavy metal toxicity from dental fillings, and contaminated food and water also add to your total toxic load. Even prolonged mental stress and negative emotions, as we will see, can create internal poisons. Lack of exercise can contribute to toxicity, too. As the body's natural cleansing cycle of oxygen and vital nutrients depend upon exercise, a stagnant system encourages toxic build-up, like a clogged drainpipe.

Your body does have protective measures in place. It surrounds these potentially dangerous toxins with mucus or fat so they won't cause an imbalance or trigger an immune reaction. This alone is a significant reason to keep your diet and body fat low: it's believed that some people carry around up to six kilograms of fat that harbours their toxic waste!

Toxins absorbed by the body are stored in your cells where they lower vitality, encourage the development of degenerative diseases and speed up the ageing process. They affect every system and organ of your body. And since your skin is a gauge for what's happening internally, it can show signs of toxic build-up.

Along with your kidneys and intestines, your skin also plays a major role in detoxification; it's responsible for eliminating cellular waste and functions as a backup for other elimination organs. If your colon becomes stagnant with toxins or your liver can't efficiently filter impurities from your digestive tract, your skin tries to compensate by releasing the toxins. It sweats them out or throws them off through rashes, acne and boils. Eliminated toxins also show themselves as pimples, uneven skin texture and unnaturally oily or unbalanced skin.

Obviously, it isn't practical to completely avoid all toxins, so the next best thing is to keep pollutants and toxins to a minimum by periodically releasing them through a detoxification program. That is why gentle detoxification is so powerful in achieving great looking skin: it helps to get rid of accumulated toxins in your body and helps bring your skin into peak condition.

So you think you don't need a detox? Flip to the middle of the chapter and do the detox quiz. You may be surprised at how many seemingly unrelated symptoms can indicate toxicity in overdrive.

Detox diets

There are tons of detox diets, but no matter which one you choose, make sure you follow the three main elements of a good detox program:

- cleansing
- rebuilding
- maintaining.

To cleanse, you can do a modified juice detox or cut certain foods or substances — such as red meat, sugar, salt, processed foods, alcohol, caffeine or cigarettes — from your diet for a specified period. The second step of detoxification is to rebuild your system by gradually reintroducing certain foods into your diet. The third step is maintaining the positive changes you've made to your diet and lifestyle. The maintenance step is your 30-day Gorgeous Skin program.

Why not a water fast?

Some detox diets involve fasting, or an all-liquid diet. A few days without solid food can be an enlightening experience! A traditional fast generally means only water, but these days fresh juice fasts are far more common. Fresh juices — juicing at home is preferable to store-bought juices — deeply cleanse your body, rejuvenate your cells and tissues and help your body clean out its waste deposits more efficiently than water fasting. Fresh juices are easy on your digestion: they're assimilated into your bloodstream without effort, and they don't disturb the detoxification process. Vegetable and fruit juices are also alkalising, so they neutralise uric acid and other inorganic acids better than water. Juices better support improved metabolic activity for fasting, which ensures productive cleansing; during a water fast, as your body attempts to conserve dwindling energy resources, metabolic activity slows down.

I generally don't recommend a water fast because it can be too harsh and demanding on your body. And sometimes the physical and emotional stress of a water fast overrides the healing benefits. Today, with large amounts of environmental toxins around, it can even be dangerous. Because many toxins are fat-soluble and are stored in fat cells, these buried pollutants and chemicals can be released into your elimination channels too rapidly. Then, when your cells burn fat, they also release the toxic substances they've been storing. As toxin levels in the blood increase, so does the risk of serious damage to tissues; your body is essentially re-poisoned as the chemicals move through your bloodstream.

Detox away skin disorders

A great detox can work wonders for almost any skin condition. Nutritionists and naturopaths have used elimination diets and detox programs to treat various skin problems for years. This is because faulty detoxification mechanisms, too many toxins, and an over-worked liver can aggravate many skin conditions such as acne, acne rosacea, skin healing, psoriasis, eczema, dermatitis, cellulite, rashes, hives, cold sores, fungal infections, facial puffiness, impetigo, vitiligo and warts.

Poor digestion and allergies can exacerbate these as well. And a compromised liver function can trigger or provoke allergic skin conditions. Optimising detoxification and digestion, as well as addressing any suspected food allergies, is a powerful way to treat a variety of skin conditions without having to resort to drugs that have myriad side effects. If you do have any of the skin conditions above, you are sure to benefit from the detox program under the supervision of a qualified health professional (remember, dermatologists generally aren't trained in areas of nutrition, allergies or environmental medicine). If you do suspect allergies, consider an elimination or rotation diet, again under the supervision of your health care practitioner.

Detoxification for gorgeous skin

Through extensive research, client feedback and my own personal experience, I've found that a brief three- or even a seven-day juice cleanse along with nutritional support is the best way to release toxins from your body. Shorter cleanses will have some benefit but you truly begin to see and feel the difference after three days. The program consists of fresh juices, raw or lightly steamed non-starchy, low-GI vegetables of your choice, at least eight glasses of filtered/spring/mineral water per day, herbal teas, a vegetable broth (see Recipes, page 264), antioxidants/herbal liver support, along with a protein powder that contains nutrients to help support detoxification. So it certainly doesn't mean you have to starve!

A three- to seven-day detox 'cleans your pipes' of systemic sludge, excess mucous, old faecal matter, trapped cellular and non-food wastes and inorganic mineral deposits! And it will jump-start your Gorgeous Skin program. Even a relatively short fast accelerates elimination, often causing dramatic changes as masses of accumulated waste are expelled. I generally don't recommend more than seven days except in a controlled, clinical environment.

But be prepared! You won't feel fantastic on the first day or two of your fast! You'll know your body is detoxing if you experience a short period of headaches, fatigue, light headedness, body odour, bad breath, a coated tongue, diarrhoea or even mouth sores that commonly accompany accelerated elimination. However, digestion usually improves straight away. Your skin may also break out, its texture may look uneven, or you may just look and feel 'blah' for the first few days. If you eliminate toxins too quickly, you run a greater risk of developing these side-effects, which is why I recommend easing into the program as you will see.

Now, let's take at look at your digestion and your liver function — the key players in detoxification. Then we'll see whether a detox program is right for you.

Digestion — your skin, the mirror

Proper digestion is one of the key elements to feeling good, preventing disease and looking youthful. Even though you may be eating healthily, nutrients and minerals will not be properly absorbed in your body without proper digestion. So to rephrase an old saying, you are not only 'what you eat', but also what you digest and what you absorb. Nutrition, digestion, absorption and your bacterial balance all play critical roles in the health of your gastrointestinal (GI) tract, your body overall, and of course, your skin. We spend huge amounts of time and effort keeping our bodies clean from the outside while doing nothing to promote and maintain healthy and clean bodies on the inside. Unfortunately, most people completely ignore their GI tract until it gives them serious problems.

But great digestion is a key step to maintaining optimal skin. As I've mentioned, from a naturopathic and nutritional perspective, the root of many chronic skin problems can be found in disturbed or compromised digestive functions. Think of your digestive system like the roots of a tree: when the roots are strong, the tree is strong. When the roots are diseased, the whole tree is diseased. The same goes for your digestive system, when functioning optimally, you will have great health and gorgeous skin.

So how do you know whether your digestive system is working optimally? Some symptoms can be very subtle, but the most obvious indicators of digestive disturbances are:

- upset stomach
- abdominal pain
- bloating
- intestinal gas
- nausea
- vomiting
- constipation

- diarrhoea
- rumbling noises (not when you're hungry)
- burning sensation after eating
- feeling particularly full after meals.

All of these symptoms can be aggravated by food allergies or sensitivities.

Tips for optimal digestion

- Eat when relaxed. When you're stressed and race through your meals, or even angry, your nervous system sends out impulses to your extremities, which shunts blood away from your digestive system.
- Avoid consuming fluids with meals; it dilutes your digestive juices. Allow at least half an hour before a meal and one hour after.
- Start a meal with bitter greens, some lemon juice in water, or a tablespoon of apple cider vinegar. These will kick-start your digestive juices.
- Chew your food slowly to mix it with saliva. Digestion actually starts in your mouth. Chew at least twenty-five times per mouthful.
- Eat only until you're 80 per cent full. The Japanese have a saying *'Hara hachi bu'*, which means to eat until you are eight parts full (out of ten). So leave a little room at the end of each meal, as it takes about twenty minutes for the stretch receptors in your stomach to tell your brain how full you really are.

With age, the production of your digestive enzymes dwindles. This leads to decreased digestion and absorption of nutrients, along with an increased accumulation of putrefied faecal matter in your intestinal tract. Undigested food material and metabolic waste can also build up due to sluggish elimination, setting the stage for various health and skin problems.

Your liver — longevity factor

Your liver is probably your hardest working organ. It has hundreds of tasks to perform, including detoxification and filtration of your blood. It also neutralises and eliminates toxins such as the contraceptive pill, alcohol, antibiotics and caffeine. And it is a reservoir for sugar and fat. In fact it's usually congested with a glut of fat and sugar, so much so that the average person, the so-called healthy person, often uses more than sixty per cent of their liver just for storage!

Another major role of the liver is to function like a filter. If your body has too many toxins or waste products to handle, the filter becomes clogged and ineffective. When toxins aren't eliminated, they can recirculate through your blood and affect many of your organ functions as described earlier.

———————————■———————————

Optimal digestion and absorption of nutrients, along with your liver's efficient processing of toxins, are absolutely critical for great health and beauty. That's why a detox program can be such a powerful tool to rejuvenate your body and your skin from the inside out. I hope you're sufficiently motivated. Now let's get into the specifics!

Sure signs of toxicity

Do you have sallow skin?	Poor skin colouring may indicate waste build-up from liver malfunction or drug residues.
Do you have age spots?	Brown mottled spots on your hands, neck, or face may reflect waste accumulation in your liver.
Do you have adult acne or an uneven skin texture?	Waste build up from environmental pollutants, poor diet, liver exhaustion, and stress allow increased free radical formation, which can attack skin cell membranes.
Do you have wrinkles or sagging skin contours?	Free radical activity also affects collagen and elastin, resulting in wrinkling and dry skin. Ditto for too many refined sugars and carbohydrates in your diet.
Do you have puffy or swollen eyes or dark circles under your eyes?	This can be a sign that your kidneys are not performing optimally and that you have an overload of fluid waste. A number of different allergies can also cause both of these.
Do you have bad breath?	Your body may not be getting rid off toxins efficiently. It can also indicate digestive disturbances.
Do you have a skin disorder such as psoriasis, dermatitis or eczema?	Skin disorders can indicate faulty detoxification mechanisms, allergies, or poor digestion.
Do you have rashes or skin sores that aren't healing?	Poor wound healing can indicate a deficiency of vitamin C or zinc or other deficiency. Rashes may also reflect allergies.

Detox quiz

Read through the following questions and rate yourself from 0 to 2.
The more 2s you score, the greater your need for a detox.

	Never	Rarely	Often
Do you feel tired, lethargic, or sluggish?	0	1	2
Do you have difficulty concentrating or have slow or fuzzy thinking?	0	1	2
Do you feel depressed or have mood swings?	0	1	2
Do you get more than two colds per year?	0	1	2
Do you get post-nasal drip, congestion, or a 'stuffed up' nose or sinuses?	0	1	2
Do you have bad breath, a coated tongue, or a bitter or metallic taste in your mouth?	0	1	2
Do you have body odour?	0	1	2
Do you have strong smelling urine?	0	1	2
Do you have trouble sleeping or wake feeling unrefreshed?	0	1	2
Do you have sore muscles or joints?	0	1	2
Are your nails weak or brittle?	0	1	2
Do you have dark circles under your eyes?	0	1	2
Do you have digestive disturbances such as bloating, gas, or indigestion a couple of hours after eating?	0	1	2
Do you have less than one bowel movement per day?	0	1	2
Do you feel anxious or stressed out?	0	1	2
Are you sensitive to odours, foods, or chemicals?	0	1	2
Do you have allergies?	0	1	2
Do you have eczema, dry skin, acne or skin rashes?	0	1	2
Do you gain weight easily?	0	1	2
Do you have food cravings?	0	1	2
Do you have pain or discomfort under your right ribcage?	0	1	2
Does dietary fibre cause constipation?	0	1	2
Do you feel like you're not as healthy as other people your age?	0	1	2

! The above symptoms can all result from a variety of medical conditions, many of which can't adequately be helped by a detoxification diet. For example, a high score on this quiz doesn't rule out
the possibility of hypothyroidism. It's important to consult a qualified health care practitioner before you begin your detoxification
program. A short detoxification program is generally safe; however, a detoxification program shouldn't be undertaken by pregnant
women, nursing mothers, children or patients with chronic degenerative diseases, cancer or tuberculosis. Consult your health care
practitioner if you have questions about whether detoxing is right
for you.

The five-day detox countdown

The key to comfortable detoxification is to *ease* yourself into the
program, so that your body doesn't go into shock.

First, lighten up your toxic load. For five days before you begin
your detox, progressively eliminate alcohol, coffee, cigarettes, refined
sugars, saturated fats, all processed and refined foods, wheat and
dairy. These can each act as toxins in your body.

Follow a wholefood diet. Eat at least five servings of vegetables
and, if possible, eat half of the servings raw as salads. Eat fruit one to three times per day. Ensure
you eat lots of mineral-rich foods such as leafy
greens, capsicums, broccoli, sesame and sunflower seeds, fish and sea vegetables.

Increase fibre to help keep your colon clean.
Along with the fibre from vegetables and fruit,
include two tablespoons of flaxseed meal, plus
whole grains (like oats and brown rice), and
beans (pinto and black beans). Fibre acts like an
internal broom, grabbing toxins and helping

 TIP

Gradually wean yourself off
caffeine for the five days
before your detox. If you go
cold turkey you'll get nasty
headaches and other with-
drawal symptoms. Replace
coffee with green or herbal
tea.

remove them from your body. Don't forget to start drinking lots of filtered or natural mineral water too — at least 8 glasses per day.

Some specific foods that are helpful in promoting detoxification include:

- good sources of water-soluble fibre such as vegetables, pears, apples, oat bran and legumes
- garlic, onions, eggs, and other foods with a high sulphur content
- cabbage family vegetables, especially broccoli, Brussels sprouts and cabbage
- artichokes, beetroot, carrots, dandelion greens and herbs and spices such as turmeric, cinnamon and liquorice.

Also, minimise the use of chemical-based household cleaners and personal health care products (cleansers, shampoos, deodorants and toothpastes), and substitute with natural alternatives.

Another deterrent to good health is stress, as it triggers your body to release stress hormones. While these hormones can provide the 'adrenaline rush' to win a race or meet a deadline, in large amounts they create toxins and slow down detoxification enzymes in your liver. It's a good idea to detox stressful life situations along with your body. Keep a diary and take note not only of what you eat and drink but also of your emotions.

Detox aids

Along with the three-day detox diet there are systemic non-dietary ways to help speed up your detox process.

Dry skin brushing

Detoxification occurs first and foremost through your lymph. Your lymph is the interstitial fluid that bathes your cells, bringing them nutrients and removing the waste. Your body contains far more lymph than blood, and yet your lymph is dependent upon outside forces for its circulation through your body. In other words, your lymph has no heart to pump it; it relies on exercise and massage for its vital circulation, two things that are often missing in most people's lives. You can prompt your body to release its toxic deposits into your lymph by using a process called dry skin brushing, which feels fantastic!

Dry skin brushing helps remove toxins during detoxification by stimulating circulation, cleaning your lymph system and increasing cell renewal. Your skin excretes more than 900 grams of waste each day and absorbs air and sunshine. Your skin breathes! And yet in most people, this vital route of detoxification is operating far below its capacity, because it's clogged with so many dead skin cells and the waste excreted from perspiring. Dry skin brushing is a simple, inexpensive way of removing this waste from your skin and breaking down old toxic deposits through its action on your lymph vessels and capillaries.

DIRECTIONS FOR DRY SKIN BRUSHING

- Use a soft-bristle brush made with natural vegetable fibres.
- Skin-brush before showering or bathing at least *once* per day and *twice* if possible.
- Start brushing at your feet and brush towards your heart, as it's important to follow the flow of your lymphatic fluid. For arms and legs, brush with an upward motion towards your trunk.
- Brush from your fingertips up to your shoulders and towards your heart. Use small strokes and gentle pressure.
- From your shoulders and back, brush from the sides to the centre.
- Brush down your neck and trunk towards your lower abdominal area.
- Brush for five minutes each day.

❗ Don't brush over acne or sores or over areas that are inflamed.

Dry skin brushing is best done before a bath or shower, and for optimal results each day during your detox program. Brushing must be done when your body is dry; this is vital to receive the benefits. And the brush, too, must be kept dry, as any exposure to water will soften its bristles and deprive your skin of its stimulating effect. The entire surface of your skin should be brushed, with the exception of any broken or cracked skin and your face, which is generally too sensitive to be brushed. Your skin may feel tender at first, but if you continue to brush on a regular basis, you'll soon feel the benefits and you'll come to crave the daily brush!

TIP

After dry skin brushing, either before or after your shower, slather your body with extra-virgin olive oil instead of your usual body moisturiser. It is a great option, because it's rich in antioxidants. Jerry Hall has been swearing by olive oil as her beauty treatment for years!

Rebounding

Another great way to help drain your lymph and speed up the removal of toxins and waste from your body is by 'rebounding', or bouncing up and down on a mini trampoline. This low-impact exercise stimulates drainage, easing waste material out of your lymphatic system. Rebounding also fires up cellular metabolism, energising your cells with fresh oxygen and nutrients. Plus, it's joint-friendly as the soft surface of the mini trampoline absorbs about eighty-five per cent of the shock. Rebounders and mini trampolines are available at specialty sports shops throughout Australia.

Contrast showers

Contrast showers are another great way to help accelerate your body's detox process. The contrast between hot and cold water increases circulation, promotes detoxification and strengthens your immune system. This helps bring nutrients, oxygen and immune cells to damaged and stressed tissues and carries away metabolic waste, inflammatory by-products and other toxic substances. Start with two minutes of hot water followed by one minute of cold water. Repeat this pattern at least once, always finishing with cold (e.g. two minutes hot, one minute cold, two minutes hot, one minute cold). Follow your dry skin brushing (see above) with contrast showers during your three-day detox. You'll feel refreshed and revitalised.

Exercise to excrete toxins

Exercise is important in the detoxification process as it gets your lungs working and your lymphatic system moving. Try to exercise at a level where you start to sweat — a point at which toxins are released naturally through the skin. Don't forget your skin is the largest organ of elimination and sweating eliminates toxins. Over-exertion, however, is counterproductive, because it can induce oxidative stress, meaning more free radicals. Brisk walking, cycling, and swimming are all excellent forms of exercise to supplement your detox program.

Saunas — sweat toxins away

Anything that promotes perspiration helps your skin move waste out of your body. Hot baths, exercise, saunas, hydrotherapy, Epsom salt soaks, and any activity that enhances circulation in the skin and lymphatic channels can have a cleansing and stimulating effect. Make sure you sweat for fifteen to thirty minutes several times per week, even daily if you can during the three days of your detox. Saunas are a wonderful way to help you achieve this. The heat of the sauna causes you to sweat and release toxins, including heavy metals.

Saunas aren't recommended for women who are pregnant though, as the heat from the sauna may cause neural tube defects in the foetus during the first trimester of pregnancy. Those with heart disease, kidney disease, or anaemia should also refrain from saunas.

Epsom salts

Epsom salts also help draw toxins out of your body. Start with a very clean bathtub, take a shower, and then fill the tub with the hottest water you can stand. Begin with a quarter cup of Epsom salts and gradually work up to four cups in successive baths. Allow yourself up to half an hour to soak in the bath. If you experience light-headedness, drain the bathtub and wait until you feel steady to stand up. Otherwise, take a shower afterwards and dry off with a clean towel. Combined with dry skin brushing, essential oils, and soothing music, an Epsom salts soak can be a luxurious yet inexpensive detox tool.

Colonics — an optional extra

From a naturopathic perspective, optimal health and gorgeous skin are also a reflection of your elimination status. A well-functioning, clean colon means efficient absorption of key nutrients and great elimination. But take a peek into the average person's colon and you'll most likely find a build-up of putrefied faecal waste on their colon wall! This build-up of undigested matter can block proper digestion, nutrient absorption and waste elimination and provide an excellent breeding ground for germs and parasites, which are then often recirculated into the blood stream and eliminated through the skin!

Colon cleansing, colon therapy, colonic irrigation, colonics and colon hydrotherapy are all different names for the same thing. The late Princess Diana of Wales, as well as many other celebrities, have made high-profile endorsements of colonics for their great health benefits. Colonics can help remove pockets of encrusted matter and assist in the elimination of bacteria, toxins, gas, mucus, parasites and other forms of cellular debris. They can prevent the reabsorption of toxins and hasten their removal from your system. They can also free up your elimination pathways and, used judiciously, are a great adjunct to any detoxification program.

Colonics involve the infusion (and outflow) of filtered water via a sterilised tube into your large intestine to give your colon a thorough cleanse. The thought makes some people cringe, but a series of treatments can gently remove the debris that has built up over long periods of time. The procedure is a wonderful regenerative: it can dramatically improve your sense of wellbeing, making you feel lighter and more energetic.

Colonics also empty your colon of current matter, which can be of great relief to constipation sufferers. As anyone who has experienced bouts of constipation knows, it isn't great for your skin! This is why colonics are sometimes referred to as the ultimate beauty treatment! But just remember, colonics can flush out beneficial bacteria too, so I recommend taking probiotics (acidophilus and a bifidus powder) before and after colonics to help reinoculate your colon with friendly bacteria.

 TIP

Women who have taken antibiotics and/or the contraceptive pill are especially susceptible to changes in the colonic environment. Ditto for women who eat a diet high in refined carbohydrates.

When your toxic load is reduced, your elimination enhanced, and your colon cleansed and its function improved, you'll experience better digestion, with a reduction of intestinal gas, greater absorption of minerals and vitamins, elimination of toxins and purification of your blood and liver as well as other organs of elimination. Your eyes will also become clearer and brighter and your skin will glow with vital health.

CHOOSING A COLON THERAPIST

- Ask your health practitioner to direct you to a good local colon therapist.
- Look under 'Alternative Health Services' in the Yellow Pages or on the Internet.
- Make sure the colon therapist you choose is properly trained and working in a spotless facility using disposable equipment and filtered water.

Detox supplements

Taking nutrients — especially antioxidants — during your detox process is an absolute must. As a group, the antioxidant nutrients protect your cells and membranes from toxins and oxidising agents. I recommend a daily dose of an excellent antioxidant formula along with the herb milk thistle to support liver detoxification and protect it from harmful toxins. A high-potency multiple vitamin and mineral supplement is also essential. Your liver, brain and immune system in particular are dependent on a high level of vitamins and minerals in order to function properly.

Another key supplement during your detoxification program is a green drink containing dehydrated barley, alfalfa and wheat grasses as well as algae sources such as chlorella or spirulina. These green superfoods are power packed full of antioxidants and phytonutrients that work to protect your cells and promote detoxification. Young barley leaves and wheat grass are great natural sources of chlorophyll, minerals (particularly magnesium, calcium and potassium), vitamins and enzymes which are all needed for the proper metabolism of cells. They also have high enzyme and antioxidant activity.

Chlorophyll is a phytonutrient that gives leaves, plants and algae their green hue. It's actually the plant equivalent of the oxygen-carrying red pigment haemoglobin in red blood cells. Chlorophyll also alkalises the pH of the blood. There's an old saying in natural medicine: 'When you are green inside, you are clean inside!' Another must on the program is a protein powder (non-allergenic) that includes vitamins, minerals and fibre, plus substances designed to boost glutathione — one of your body's key detoxification molecules. Lastly and most importantly you need to be drinking at least eight glasses of water daily during the three-day detox program to help your body carry away the toxins that you'll be releasing.

The three-day detox program

So you've done your five-day gradual detox countdown and now you're ready for your three-day detox program. Choose a stress-free, work-free time for the detox. It's best if you try to schedule it over a long weekend without parties or other social engagements. It requires discipline, not distractions!

Breaking your detox slowly and healthily is just as important too. Make sure you don't finish it with a pizza and ice-cream, or you will undo all the good work you've done! It may take a day or so until you're back in peak performance again, so make sure you don't have any major work commitments, presentations or big meetings just after you break your detox diet.

The first and second days can be the toughest, so make sure you have the full support of your friends and families. Better yet, do it with someone for moral support and encouragement. These three days are a chance to focus fully on you — physically, mentally and emotionally. Free from food, distractions, and the daily grind, it can give you an opportunity to clear out any emotional clutter or stagnation and stimulate creativity and insight. Fasting is also really beneficial when you are contemplating some sort of life change.

During these three days I highly recommend some form of a feel-good reward, such as a facial, a massage, a scrub or some other beauty treatment. Lymphatic drainage massages are also great as they stimulate your lymph flow, which can speed up the removal of cellular garbage and toxins, as we have seen. Even though lymphatic massage is incredibly gentle and relaxing, it works on a deep level to help your body detoxify. Plus, all forms of massage encourage blood flow and deliver oxygen and nutrients to your skin's surface.

DAY ONE DETOXIFICATION

Upon rising

- Drink half a lemon squeezed into a glass of warm water (lemon juice in water has a slightly laxative effect and will stimulate your liver).
- Follow with a brisk thirty-minute walk, bike ride, rebound or swim.
- Dry-brush your skin for five minutes.
- Enjoy a contrast shower (alternate with hot and cold water; see pages 182–3).

Breakfast

- Fresh juice — try carrot, apple and ginger juice or choose from the list below.

Fruits you can juice	Vegetables you can juice
apple	carrot
grape	beetroot
grapefruit	celery
orange	cucumber
kiwi	spinach
lemon	lettuce
pear	cabbage
pineapple	parsley
	wheat grass

- Mix one tablespoon of a 'green' superfood powder of choice (containing de-hydrated barley grass, wheat grass or algae sources such as chlorella or spirulina) into a glass of water or added to a mix of water and juice. (See Resources.)

Lunch

- Raw or lightly steamed vegetables (non-starchy, low-GI vegies of choice; see table, page 53).

Dinner
- Vegetable broth (page 264).
- Fresh juice — choose from the list.

Snacks
- Drink as much water, vegetable broth and unsweetened herbal tea as you wish during the day. Aim for at least eight glasses of water within the day.
- Supplements: milk thistle; a high potency vitamin and mineral supplement; plus an antioxidant formula.
- One scoop twice daily of a non-allergenic protein powder that includes vitamins, minerals and fibre plus substances designed to boost glutathione — one of your body's key detoxification molecules (see Resources, page 304).

Before bed
- Try yoga or stretching, followed by an Epsom salts bath.

DAY TWO DETOXIFICATION

Upon rising
- Drink half a lemon squeezed into a glass of warm water.
- Follow with a brisk thirty-minute walk, bike ride, rebound or swim.
- Dry-brush your skin for five minutes.
- Enjoy a contrast shower (alternate with hot and cold water).

Breakfast
- Fresh juice of your choice with one tablespoon of a 'green' powder.

Lunch
- Raw or lightly steamed vegetables (non-starchy, low-GI vegies of choice).

Dinner
- Vegetable broth.

Snacks
- Drink as much water, vegetable broth and unsweetened herbal tea as you wish during the day. Aim for at least eight glasses of water.

TIP

Today would be a great day to book some sort of beauty treatment like a facial, a lymphatic massage or a body wrap.

- Supplements: milk thistle, a high-potency vitamin and mineral supplement; plus an antioxidant formula.
- One scoop twice during the day of non-allergenic protein powder in filtered or natural spring/mineral water.

Before bed
- Do yoga, mediation or stretching.
- Dry skin brushing followed by a shower or a bath.

DAY THREE DETOXIFICATION

Upon rising
- Drink half a lemon squeezed into a glass of warm water.
- Follow with a brisk thirty-minute walk, bike ride, rebound or swim.
- Dry-brush your skin for five minutes.
- Enjoy a contrast shower.

TIP

Have a lymphatic massage or some other personal reward today.

Breakfast
Fresh juice of your choice; mix in one tablespoon of a 'green' powder.

Lunch
Raw or lightly steamed vegetables (non-starchy, low-GI vegies of choice).

Dinner
Vegetable broth (page 264).

Snacks
- Drink as much water, vegetable broth and unsweetened herbal tea as you wish during the day. Aim for at least eight glasses of water during the day.
- Supplements: milk thistle; a high-potency vitamin and mineral supplement; plus an antioxidant formula.
- One scoop twice daily of non-allergenic protein powder in water.

Before bed
- Do yoga or stretching.
- Soak in an Epsom salt tub.

8

The 30-Day Countdown

The Gorgeous Skin Program

Having reached this point you are probably thinking: I really want to look and feel great, but how could I possibly remember all of the things that I need to do? Not to worry ... this chapter puts together all the principles that we've discussed for achieving lifelong health and beauty into a complete 30-day diet and lifestyle program! And the best part is you won't have to remember a thing, as every page is packed with detailed meal plans and reminders and tips. All you need to do is refer to one easy-to-follow page per day!

As you flip through these next pages, you'll see that this is not a restricted eating plan and it certainly doesn't require that you go hungry or give up everything you love to eat. Nor does it advocate a huge change of lifestyle or a rigorous exercise routine. The good news is that you can gear it towards your exact lifestyle, and if you follow the fundamentals of the program you won't have to count kilojoules, portion sizes or carbohydrate grams, or keep track of each snack along the way.

You'll discover that each meal contains a balance of quality-protein, non-starchy, low-GI carbohydrates and generous amounts of good fats. This ensures stable blood sugar and insulin levels, along with balanced hormone levels — major keys to youthful, radiant skin. Plus, every meal contains a powerhouse of anti-ageing antioxidants and plant phytonutrients such as carotenoids and flavonoids, which help fight free radicals and inflammation (major contributors to accelerated ageing), and lots of good fats to give your skin a glow.

For most people, it takes at least three to four weeks for any new lifestyle change to become a real habit. You'll start seeing great results much earlier, but try to follow the program faithfully for the full thirty days, and you'll be rewarded with greater energy, improved overall health and a rejuvenated long-term glow. But even if you do slip up occasionally (no one is perfect!), I promise you'll still reap the beauty and health benefits.

Getting ready

The Gorgeous Skin program is not about eating light; it's about eating well. Convenience and planning are vital keys to following the program and achieving great results. You'll find a shopping list at the end of this chapter. I recommend that you sit down with a pen and paper and make a weekly menu plan and shopping list. That way, you'll be certain to have all the food you need on hand.

If at all possible, cook meals that you can enjoy over several days. You'll notice that some of the recipes (especially the chicken and fish) have been designed so that you can add the leftovers to your salad the next day. If you are in the workforce, leave some time before work to organise the foods you'll cook for dinner in order to shorten preparation time when you return home. Sometimes waiting to cook a meal can trigger the nibbles. Keep chopped raw vegetables on hand for any 'pre-meal munchies'. Dip them in hummus or raw almond butter for an extra nutrient boost and to keep you going during meal preparation.

Now is the time for a big kitchen cleanout! All of those high-carbohydrate treats and foods hiding in the cupboards will call out to you at some point in time. Throw out all of these foods, including sugar, biscuits, chocolate (except the good-quality dark bittersweet kind), crackers, chips, breakfast cereals, white flour, white pasta and anything refined to stave off temptation during your program.

Also banish the bad fats, including highly refined cooking oils like corn and safflower, along with margarine. Stock up on the fabulous face fats: cold-pressed extra-virgin olive oil and macadamia nut oil.

Program guidelines

- Start each morning with either half a lemon squeezed into warm water or a cleansing herb tea.
- You can get as creative as you like with the food from the approved lists.
- Say good-bye to empty-kilojoule, sugar laden foods including soft drinks, ice-cream, anything that contains sucrose or high-fructose corn syrup, and artificial sweeteners.
- Cut out all refined grains such as white flours, breads, white rice, pastas, rice cakes, biscuits, crackers and cakes.
- Drink at least eight glasses of pure water per day. To make it more palatable squeeze in a little lime or lemon juice, or add a splash of unsweetened cranberry or apple juice or a little mint.
- Aim for as many servings of low-GI fruits and vegetables as possible every day (see table page 53), and make a point of eating different types and colours. Have at least one salad per day with dark-green leaves. With another meal steam, sauté or grill vegetables as a side dish to fish or meat.
- Make sure you are eating raw food every day. Start your meal with a little raw food to get your enzymes going and your digestive system primed.

- Eat lots of cold-water varieties of fish; aim for at least four servings per week.
- Use olive oil as your primary cooking oil. Cold-pressed coconut and cold-pressed macadamia nut oils are your next best cooking oils.
- Avoid all commercial cooking oils such as corn, safflower, sunflower and soybean oil, as well as vegetable shortening, margarine and partially hydrogenated oils.
- Use herbs (fresh and dried) and spices to flavour your foods.
- Limit your intake of dairy foods except for a small amount of natural yoghurt, feta (from goat's or sheep's milk) or hard Parmesan.
- Avoid all alcohol, especially spirits, white wine and beer, except for the occasional glass of red wine.
- Snack on seeds, nuts and snacks from the allowable snack list only.
- Wherever possible buy organic.
- Chew each mouthful slowly, focusing on your food, and eat until only about three-quarters full.
- Don't eat when stressed, upset or angry.
- To keep blood sugar levels stable, don't go longer than four hours without eating.
- Always eat protein with every meal, including breakfast. This balances out blood sugar levels and will stop you reaching for a sugary snack. And always start your meal with protein — say, fish before a soup — so it doesn't shock your system into pumping out too much insulin.
- Eat with enjoyment and savour every mouthful! Most people with weight problems don't eat with pleasure. They stuff food into their mouths like it's something to pass time, or out of pure boredom.
- Last of all, try to follow the program as faithfully as possible — that way you'll get the best results.
- What you eat today, you wear tomorrow — and not just on your hips!

Meal guidelines
Breakfast

During the 30-day program, breakfast is an absolute must to keep your blood sugar levels on an even keel. If you're not big on breakfast or don't have much time in the morning, have some yoghurt with fruit, nuts, seeds or freshly ground flaxseeds or a simple smoothie. You also must include some form of protein. Remember keeping your insulin levels low is a major key to achieving gorgeous skin.

During the week, when a lack of time tends to be an issue, you'll see that the options are easier to prepare. The Saturday and Sunday breakfast choices are based on more preparation time. So if you do feel adventurous, whip up a Gorgeous Skin Japanese breakfast of grilled salmon, miso soup and a few slices of fresh fruit.

Lunch

Vegies, vegies and more vegies! Try to eat at least one salad a day, preferably made with dark green leafy vegetables such as cos lettuce or spinach. Remember, the darker the colour of the vegetable, the higher the phytonutrient antioxidant content. In just one serving of vegetables there are more than one hundred different phytonutrients. So the more phytonutrients you eat in fruit and vegetable form, the stronger your antioxidant protection.

Feel free to get as creative as you like with the foods on the allowed lists and remember to incorporate as many colours and varieties of vegetables as possible into your salads. Include tomatoes, grated carrot and other vegetables such as cucumbers, raw sliced mushrooms, capsicums, sliced radishes, chopped parsley and celery. Add some protein such as grilled free-range chicken, fish (cooked salmon/sardines/mackerel in olive oil), eggs, tofu or prawns to your salad. Crumbled feta, avocado, toasted pine nuts, sesame seeds and walnuts make tasty and nutritious additions. Sprinkle your salads with freshly ground flax seeds for a fatty acid boost.

Cut out commercial salad dressings while you're on the program. Most dressings are made with cheap, refined oils such as safflower, soybean, sunflower, cottonseed and corn oils, which are high in Omega-6 fatty acids. Too many of these Omega-6 oils, especially the less expensive, highly refined ones, can increase free-radical activity and inflammation. Make up your own dressing with extra-virgin olive oil and a squeeze of fresh lemon juice or balsamic or red wine vinegar and fresh herbs like basil, coriander or parsley to taste. To give your dressings zest, add a crushed clove of garlic. Make it in advance so you can also take it with you to work.

Dinner

If you like to cook, indulge your creativity with fresh fish, free-range chicken and the approved low-GI non-starchy vegetables, whole grains, legumes, herbs and spices from the table at the end of this chapter. If time is an issue, or the recipes look too complicated, a great piece of fish such as salmon, cooked correctly, needs very little else. Simply brush it with a little olive oil, salt and pepper, grill and serve with freshly chopped herbs. Steam, grill or sauté vegetables such as spinach, broccoli, cauliflower, asparagus, beetroot, eggplant and green beans as a side dish. A little garlic, olive oil, lemon and fresh herbs will enhance the flavour of almost any vegetable. If you crave extra carbohydrates, serve with some organic brown or wild rice.

Please keep red meat to a minimum during the program. Most commercially raised meats tend to be high in saturated fat, plus they can contain antibiotics, hormones, pesticides, preservatives, and colouring agents — all toxins that sabotage your health and ultimately your skin. The natural and synthetic hormones found in meat can upset our delicate hormonal systems. Also, these days cattle and many other domesticated livestock are typically fed cereal grains (such as corn) for several months before slaughter, increasing their overall fat, saturated fat and pro-inflammatory Omega-6 fatty acid content. So eat only small portions of the leanest cuts, from grass fed and certified organically raised cattle where possible.

Snacks

This is the most challenging area for people to make appropriate choices. It's so easy to stray from the program when choosing drinks, snacks and desserts, but this will undo all your good work and set you back in your pursuit of gorgeous skin. So if you do feel hungry between meals, stick to foods on the allowable snack list. Each choice is loaded with antioxidants, vitamins, minerals, good fats and phytonutrients for gorgeous skin.

Raw unsalted nuts and seeds such as almonds, cashews, macadamias, walnuts, pistachios, and pumpkin seeds make a great in-between meal snack. They're filled with plenty of essential fats, minerals such as magnesium for beautiful skin, plus they balance out blood sugar levels and keep you satisfied for longer. If you are trying to lose weight you'll want to limit your intake of nuts to 100 grams or less a day. See the following list for plenty of other tasty snack suggestions.

Gorgeous skin snacks

Note: Italics indicate a recipe in Chapter 10.
- Wedges of organic apples dipped in raw organic almond butter
- Half a dozen green or black olives
- Raw almonds/raw unsalted macadamia nuts/raw walnuts
- Low-GI fruits, such as pears and apples

- Bowl of fresh blackberries or blueberries sprinkled with almond slices
- Half a cup of frozen red grapes (in hot weather)
- *Roasted soy nuts*
- Raspberry–mango elixir: fresh chilled raspberries or blueberries, 1 medium chilled mango, vanilla soymilk, natural yoghurt with a small amount of raw honey (whiz ingredients together in a blender)
- Edamame (whole green soybeans boiled in their skins for ten minutes in salty water)
- Raw vegies (green capsicum strips, cherry tomatoes, sliced cucumbers, celery or carrots) dipped in nut butters like almond or hummus (see *Creamy hummus dip*) or *Vegetable and herb tofu dip*
- Freshly juiced fruit and vegetable juices such as carrot, celery, ginger and apple
- Make your own trail mix of almonds, pistachios, pumpkin seeds, macadamias, sunflower seeds, and organic raisins (2 tablespoons at a time)
- Two figs with half a dozen almonds
- Hard-boiled organic egg
- *Whey protein blueberry shake*
- Two prunes or plums (when in season)
- Half a cup natural yoghurt (no added sugar) with fruit and raw nuts
- Half a free-range chicken breast
- Handful of sunflower seeds
- A cup of cherries
- *Almond, coconut and banana power muffins*
- Six organic dried apricots with half a dozen raw nuts, such as almonds or walnuts

Sweeteners

It may sound surprising, but this program is not about saying good-bye to all things sweet. The key is to make the correct sweetening choices and to find satisfying sugar substitutes. If you do need to sweeten up your life a bit from time to time (as we all do!), stevia, xylitol or a small amount of raw, unheated organic honey are all great choices.

Xylitol can easily be used in hot and cold beverages, in cooking, and in some baking recipes as a substitute for sugar. Chewing gum with xylitol after a meal has numerous health benefits. Besides satisfying your sweet tooth, research has shown xylitol to prevent tooth decay and even remineralise teeth![83] (See Resources, page 304, for where to purchase xylitol products.)

Organic honey contains skin-friendly phytonutrients including antioxidant-rich flavonoids.[84] The darker the honey, the higher the antioxidant content. Manuka honey is preferable as it doesn't raise insulin levels as much as other types of honey, plus it has anti-viral and anti-bacterial properties. Heating it will, however, cause the loss of these beneficial actions.

If you crave something sweet, have a small amount of fruit following your meal. Try a slice or two of rockmelon, pawpaw with lime juice, or some mixed berries. Or opt for a bowl of strawberries, raspberries, blackberries, red currants and black currants. Grill a few fresh figs with macadamia nuts and serve with fresh ricotta. You can also finish a meal with a few organic dates. Make sure you don't eat dates on an empty stomach though, as they are sky high on the GI index and will send your blood sugar levels through the roof. Stuff dates with raw almonds to blunt your blood sugar response.

During the program you can indulge in a couple of pieces of dark bittersweet chocolate every week. Dark chocolate is actually full of flavonoids — and it won't raise blood sugar levels. What you need to look for is a high-quality semi-sweet or bittersweet chocolate with seventy per cent or more pure cocoa (organic if possible) (see the Resources section). Avoid all white and milk chocolates; they have none of the benefits of the dark variety — they're just pure sugar, fat and empty kilojoules.

Alcohol and caffeine

As mentioned above, you'll be asked to forgo alcohol during the 30 days, especially white wine, spirits and beer. However, you can enjoy up to three glasses of red wine per week as a special treat. Just make sure you don't drink them on an empty stomach (always with food) or all in one sitting!

If you absolutely can't kick your caffeine, try to cut back to a maximum of three cups of coffee per week. Make sure it's good espresso coffee (not the filtered variety as filtered coffee is, surprisingly, much higher in caffeine) and down a glass of water with each cup to make up for its dehydrating effects. Also brewed coffee kept on a warming plate should be avoided as it accelerates oxidation. But don't drink it on an empty stomach, as this will send your pro-inflammatory stress hormone levels through the roof.

Just 400 grams of your favourite coffee contains enough caffeine to raise your adrenaline level by more than two hundred per cent; pump out enough adrenaline and your cortisol levels rise. In fact, three cups of coffee a day can cause your blood cortisol levels to stay high for about eighteen of the twenty-four hours, in contrast with the usual few hours for which cortisol is supposed to be elevated! Remember: as cortisol rises, your body's level of DHEA — your 'youth hormone' — decreases. Better yet, trade your usual cup of coffee for antioxidant-rich green tea, herbal tea or some hot water with a squeeze of lemon. Your skin will thank you!

Beauty drinks

- Water with a squeeze or wedge of lemon, orange, lime or mint
- Sparkling mineral water with a splash of apple, grapefruit, orange, unsweetened cranberry juice or grape juice and a twist of lime
- Green tea
- Fresh juices (diluted with water)
- Herbal tea (loose or in bags, organic if possible)
- Freshly juiced vegetable and low-GI fruit juices such as carrot, tomato, apple, pear, lemon, ginger, beetroot and celery
- Unsweetened chai tea
- Dandelion/soy coffee
- Whey/soy smoothies
- Teeccino herbal coffees — made from a blend of herbs, grains, fruits and nuts that are roasted and ground to brew and taste just like coffee. (See Resources.)

Gorgeous skin while dining out

The Gorgeous Skin program is designed to be practical and user friendly, so even dining out will be a breeze. In Australia, we're blessed with great seafood, fresh vegetables and an abundance of super-healthy foods. If you are going out with friends, steer them to a restaurant where you can make healthy choices like fish and a fresh salad.

Modern Australian and Mediterranean-style cuisine are your best bets when eating out. Fish, chicken and vegetables should be grilled, roasted, steamed or poached rather than fried. Opt for a piece of grilled fish or free-range chicken, a salad with a simple dressing of olive oil and balsamic vinegar, and some non-starchy, low-GI vegetables such as mushrooms, asparagus or green beans. Just steer clear of pastas, breads and potatoes — and, of course, sauces and anything fried. You can also go for Middle Eastern, Greek or Japanese cuisine.

Just forgo the white rice and noodles as these increase the glycaemic load of a meal. Also beware of many sauces like teriyaki, which are loaded with sugar. When in doubt, always ask. Chinese food should generally be avoided, as many dishes tend to be stir-fried in oils that are high in pro-inflammatory fats like soybean, and they often contain MSG and a whole host of other skin baddies.

Before your restaurant meal enjoy a glass of water with a twist of lemon or lime. You can enjoy the occasional glass of red wine. However, spirits, white wine and (worst of all) beer should all be avoided. Soft drinks are a pure sugar rush and are a definite no-no during the 30 days.

The most sabotaging part of the restaurant meal is the bread basket. Typically you arrive and you're hungry, and there it is: that tempting, crusty and often fragrant bread being placed before you. But bread is loaded with bad carbohydrates and will jolt your bloodstream with glucose on an empty stomach. If you absolutely can't resist, ask for a little wholegrain dark rye or pumpernickel bread and dip it in virgin olive oil, which will slow down absorption of the starches and give you a feeling of fullness.

The 30-day Gorgeous Skin program

In the following pages you'll find four weeks' worth of daily menu plans, scheduled times for supplements and suggested exercise. A menu item in italics indicates that the recipe is included in Chapter 10. Feel free to mix and match from the lists of allowed foods and meal suggestions or interchange the dinner and lunch menus and to modify the recipes to suit your taste buds. As long as you stick to the basic guidelines, you'll get great results. Just remember, make sure each meal contains some great-quality protein, non-starchy low-GI carbohydrates and good fats.

Along with your Gorgeous Skin eating and supplement program, make sure you experience the luxury of deep, restful sleep, relax with yoga and meditation and do some form of exercise daily.

I highly recommend that you keep a journal during the 30 days to note your progress. You may wish to record your reactions, feelings, energy levels and the condition of your skin. Once you see the changes to your appearance, you'll have the positive reinforcement to stick to the program. Also, when you feel tempted to stray from the program, maintaining a journal can help to keep your motivation on track.

Try Zoning

I'm a big fan of the Zone style of eating pioneered by Dr Barry Sears. It's an excellent way to balance out your blood sugar levels and prevent that age-accelerating spike in insulin after meals. It's also relatively simple to follow. The basis of the Zone is to maintain balanced ratios of carbohydrates to protein and fat, which in turn keep blood sugar, as well as insulin levels, in check.

In the ideal Zone way of eating, each snack or meal should have the following ratios: about 40 per cent carbohydrates (low glycaemic), 30 per cent protein and 30 per cent fat. An easy way to ensure these ratios is to visualise the following on your plate: about one third of your plate (or about the size and thickness of your palm) should be protein; the remaining two-thirds should be low-GI carbohydrates such as asparagus, broccoli, spinach, zucchini, brown rice or lentils. Add some nuts or olive oil for the fat content and you have a meal that's approximately in the Zone. Not only does the Zone way of eating help control your insulin levels but it will also help you stabilise your body weight by helping you burn your own body fat, balance out energy levels and stay satisfied for longer!

SYMBOLS

Weight training

Aerobic exercise

Supplements

Relaxation yoga/meditation

DAY 1: MONDAY

BREAKFAST

- ³/₄ cup of natural yoghurt with sliced fresh fruit (choose one or mix in rockmelon, honeydew, berries, peaches, plums or pears). Sprinkle with sliced almonds or walnuts and drizzle with a little raw honey to sweeten if desired. Add two tablespoons of freshly ground flax seeds.
- Green tea/herbal tea

LUNCH

- Salad of lettuce, rocket, tomatoes, mushrooms, fresh herbs, crumbled goat's cheese, slices of pears and chopped walnuts. Drizzle with extra-virgin olive oil, balsamic vinegar and lemon juice.
- 1 tin canned salmon in brine/water/spring water
- 1 slice of wholegrain dark rye or pumpernickel bread

DINNER

- Grilled salmon steak with a *Greek salad* (save some salmon for your salad tomorrow)
- 2 slices rockmelon along with a few raw unsalted macadamia nuts

THROUGHOUT THE DAY

- Snacks mid-morning/afternoon (from snack list)
  Weight training

The Greek wrinkle cure! Dose up on at least two table-spoons of olive oil a day this week for smooth, supple skin.

DAY 2: TUESDAY

BREAKFAST

- Slow-cooked (not instant) oatmeal with fresh apples and cinnamon, or with mixed berries. Toss in the fruit during the last few minutes of the cooking time to warm it while still preserving freshness and flavour. Add some crushed walnuts and serve with soy milk, rice milk, almond milk or coconut cream/milk.
- Green tea/herbal tea
- Skin supplements

LUNCH

- A baby spinach salad, with vine-ripened tomatoes, green and red capsicums, broccoli florets, Spanish onion, grated carrot and cooked flaked salmon (from the night before); handful of almonds
- Skin supplements

DINNER

- Free-range chicken (without skin) and cashews sautéed in olive oil with fresh garlic, and organic tamari (wheat-free soy sauce). Serve with a salad of watercress and sliced cucumbers, broccoli and grated carrot and tossed with virgin olive oil and balsamic vinegar.
- Fresh blackberries and raspberries or any other low-GI fruit in season.

THROUGHOUT THE DAY

Snack mid-morning/afternoon (from the snack list)

- Some form of aerobic exercise, e.g. running, swimming
- Daily relaxation 20 minutes

DAY 3: WEDNESDAY

BREAKFAST

- Half an avocado mashed on a piece of wholegrain rye toast, drizzled with a little olive oil and pepper
- Soft-boiled egg
- 2 slices of rockmelon
- Skin supplements

LUNCH

- *Asparagus and lentil salad with tomato–lemon dressing*
- Small pear or apple
- Skin supplements

DINNER

- *Roasted ocean trout with pesto crust*
- Steamed spinach and broccoli
- Mixed green salad with avocado, fresh herbs, garlic, extra-virgin olive oil, fresh lemon juice or balsamic vinegar
- 2 dried figs, half a dozen almonds

THROUGHOUT THE DAY

Snack mid-morning/afternoon (from the snack list)

- Some form of aerobic exercise or weight training
- Daily relaxation 20 minutes

Elevate your head. Propping your head up with an extra pillow reduces eye puffiness that can add years to your face. Gravity drains fluid so it doesn't pool around your eyes.

DAY 4: THURSDAY

BREAKFAST

- *Whey protein blueberry shake*
- Skin supplements

LUNCH

- Grilled chicken on a bed of lettuce, tomatoes, cucumbers, sliced radish, green capsicum, avocado and walnuts. Dress with olive oil and lemon juice.
- 1 serving of low-GI fruit
- Skin supplements

DINNER

- *Gazpacho*
- Yellow-fin tuna grilled and seasoned with fresh garlic and freshly ground pepper
- Steamed mixed vegetables (broccoli, cauliflower, spinach, red capsicums or other low-GI vegies) tossed with virgin olive oil, lemon juice and garlic
- *Baked peaches with ricotta*
- Think colour! Try to eat as many deeply and vibrantly coloured fruits and vegetables as possible for the next few weeks.

THROUGHOUT THE DAY

Snack mid-morning/afternoon (from the snack list)

- Some form of aerobic exercise or weight training
- Daily relaxation 20 minutes

Get energised! Droopy eyelids and non-stop yawning are hardly hallmarks of youthful exuberance. For a safe natural lift, take Siberian Ginseng (*Eleutherococcus senticosus*) in capsule or liquid form.

DAY 5: FRIDAY

BREAKFAST

- Make a fruit compote of dried prunes, apricots, peaches, and apples pre-soaked in mineral water and sprinkled with flaked almonds and two tablespoons of ground flax seeds. Serve with soy or goat's milk yoghurt. Add two tablespoons of whey protein powder.
- Green tea/herbal tea
- Skin supplements

LUNCH

- *Avocado and rocket salad with basil–mustard vinaigrette*
- Small can of sardines/mackerel/salmon in olive oil or water
- Handful of macadamia nuts
- Skin supplements

DINNER

- *Steamed snapper with ginger and shallots*
- Steamed (low-GI) vegetables of choice with fresh herbs, drizzled with olive oil and crushed pumpkin seeds
- 1/2 cup organic brown or wild rice
- 2 slices of rockmelon

THROUGHOUT THE DAY

Snack mid-morning/afternoon (from the snack list)

- Some form of aerobic exercise or weight training
- Daily relaxation 20 minutes

> Move with grace. If you don't move well, you'll look old, now matter how gorgeous your figure, hair or makeup is. And don't slouch!

DAY 6: SATURDAY

BREAKFAST

- *Prawn and avocado omelette*
- Orange and honeydew slices on the side
- Green tea/herbal tea
- Skin supplements

LUNCH

- Salad of fresh spinach with thinly sliced (free-range) chicken or turkey. Add strips of red capsicum, slices of fresh mushrooms and onion. Sprinkle sunflower seeds over the salad. Toss with virgin olive oil, lemon and fresh herbs.
- Skin supplements

DINNER

- *Barramundi with lime, ginger and shiitake mushrooms*
- Steamed asparagus and string beans
- 1/2 cup brown rice
- *Grilled fresh figs with macadamia nuts and ricotta*

THROUGHOUT THE DAY

Snack mid-morning/afternoon (from the snack list)

- Some form of aerobic exercise or weight training
- Daily relaxation 20 minutes

DAY 7: SUNDAY

BREAKFAST

- Japanese breakfast of grilled salmon, *miso vegetable soup*, sliced tomatoes and Spanish onion salad, sprinkled with olive oil and vinegar
- 2 slices of rockmelon
- Green tea/herbal tea
- Skin supplements

LUNCH

- *Lentil and vegetable soup*
- Serve with tossed greens, dressed with olive oil and a splash of lemon juice.
- Handful of raw almonds, pecans and raisins
- Skin supplements

DINNER

- *Grilled chicken breasts with mushrooms* (served with wild rice)
- Steamed green beans and a salad of dark leafy greens
- Compote of prunes, apricots and berries

THROUGHOUT THE DAY

Snack mid-morning/afternoon (from the snack list)

- Daily relaxation 20 minutes

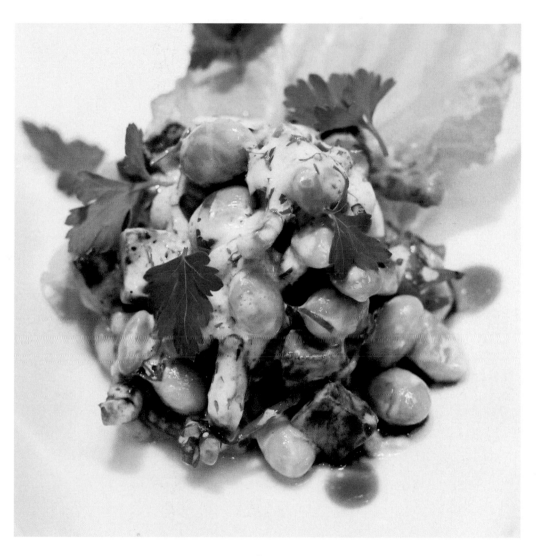

Get your protein, phytonutrients and antioxidants
all in one from the **Edamame salad**.

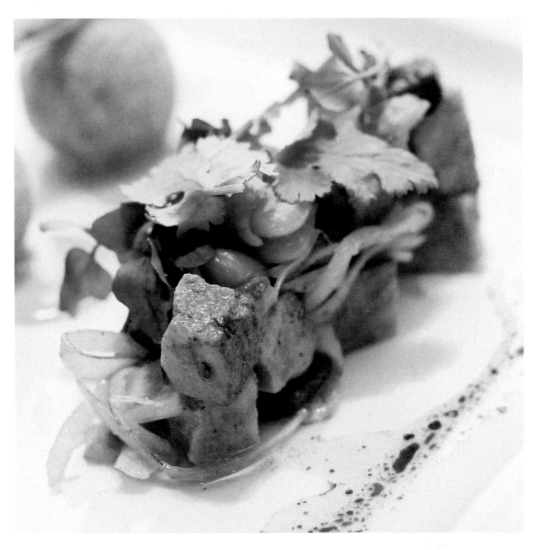

Balance your blood sugar levels
with the luscious **Moroccan beef salad**.

DAY 8: MONDAY

BREAKFAST

- *Scrambled tofu*, piece of wholegrain rye or gluten-free toast
- Green tea/herbal tea
- Skin supplements

LUNCH

- Sardines in olive oil with a tossed salad of dark leafy greens, avocado, walnuts, grated carrots, onion and tomatoes. Drizzle with olive oil, balsamic vinegar and lemon juice.
- 1 apple or 1 pear
- Handful of raw unsalted nuts
- Skin supplements

DINNER

- *Grilled salmon (fillets or steaks) with chilli coriander pesto*
- Steamed broccoli, snow peas and a large green salad
- 2 slices of rockmelon

THROUGHOUT THE DAY

Snack mid-morning/afternoon (from the snack list)
- Some form of aerobic exercise or weight training
- Daily relaxation 20 minutes

Act young. If you simply believe you're young and behave youthfully, you'll look and feel the part.

DAY 9: TUESDAY

BREAKFAST

- *Cavewoman muesli*, add half a grated apple or a handful of berries (fresh or frozen), and serve with soymilk, almond milk, rice milk or coconut cream/milk
- Green tea/herbal tea
- Skin supplements

LUNCH

- Can of sardines or salmon, served on a bed of dark leafy greens, sliced tomatoes and cucumbers, asparagus, onions, toasted pine nuts and fresh herbs
- *Tahini dressing*
- Serving of fresh low-GI fruit from recommended list
- Skin supplements

DINNER

- *Grilled red snapper with tomato salsa*
- *Sweet potato mash*
- Green salad
- 1/2 cup brown or wild rice
- Small fruit salad of low-GI fruits with natural yoghurt

THROUGHOUT THE DAY

Snack mid-morning/afternoon (from the snack list)

- Some form of aerobic exercise or weight training
- Daily relaxation 20 minutes

Get sweaty. It helps your skin flush toxins that make it look dull and blotchy. Plus, it brings fresh nutrients and oxygen to your skin.

DAY 10: WEDNESDAY

BREAKFAST
- Egg-white omelette with *salsa*
- Serving of seasonal fruits (stick to low-GI fruits such as apples, pears, peaches or berries)
- Green tea/herbal tea
- Skin supplements

LUNCH
- *Chickpea and broccoli salad with flax seed–tahini dressing*
- Handful of raisins and raw nuts
- Skin supplements

DINNER
- *Grilled miso salmon*
- ½ cup of organic brown rice
- Salad of baby spinach, avocado and toasted pine nuts
- *Mixed fresh berries with ginger sauce*

THROUGHOUT THE DAY
Snack mid-morning/afternoon (from the snack list)
- Some form of aerobic exercise or weight training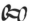
- Daily relaxation 20 minutes

DAY 11: THURSDAY

BREAKFAST

- *Fruit and nut breakfast*, served with rice milk, coconut cream/milk or natural organic yoghurt
- Green tea/herbal tea
- Skin supplements

LUNCH

- Sliced fresh turkey breast on a bed of lettuce, tomatoes, cucumbers, sliced radish and green capsicum dressed with olive oil, lemon and fresh herbs
- One serving of fruit and a handful of raw nuts
- Skin supplements

DINNER

- Fresh grilled fish of choice over rocket with sliced tomatoes, thick-sliced onions and black olives. Toss salad with a dressing of olive oil, red wine vinegar and a little fresh garlic
- *Borscht*
- Sliced apples with *almond cream*

THROUGHOUT THE DAY

Snack mid-morning/afternoon (from the snack list)

- Some form of aerobic exercise or weight training
- Daily relaxation 20 minutes

DAY 12: FRIDAY

BREAKFAST

- Poached free-range egg on wholegrain rye toast
- Baked tomato with olive oil and basil
- Green tea/herbal tea
- Skin supplements

LUNCH

- Grilled chicken breast
- Avocado salad with 1/2 small avocado, lime juice, cucumbers, spring greens, tomatoes and shallots with 1 tablespoon *flax seed dressing*
- One serving of fruit
- Skin supplements

DINNER

- Grilled prawns with *Thai-style fish sauce*
- 1/2 cup brown rice
- Wok-fried asparagus, broccoli and snow peas

THROUGHOUT THE DAY

Snack mid-morning/afternoon (from the snack list)

- Some form of aerobic exercise or weight training ♡
- Daily relaxation 20 minutes

DAY 13: SATURDAY

BREAKFAST

- ¹/₂ grapefruit
- *Spinach frittata with tomato salsa*
- Green tea/herbal tea
- Skin supplements

LUNCH

- *Beetroot and rocket salad with lemon–ginger dressing*
- 1 serving of fruit
- 2 dried figs and half a dozen raw nuts
- Skin supplements

DINNER

- Grilled snapper with herbs, olive oil and lemon OR
- *Moroccan beef salad*
- *Spinach and egg salad* with sprouts, mushrooms and radishes
- *Spicy fruit compote* with natural yoghurt or *almond cream*

THROUGHOUT THE DAY

Snack mid-morning/afternoon (from the snack list)

- Some form of aerobic exercise or weight training
- Daily relaxation 20 minutes

DAY 14: SUNDAY

BREAKFAST

- *Scrambled tofu*
- 2 slices of honeydew or rockmelon
- Skin supplements

LUNCH

- Salmon salad made with blanched green beans, Kalamata olives, capers, red onions, garlic and fresh oregano. Olive oil and balsamic vinegar dressing.
- 1 serving of fruit
- Skin supplements

DINNER

- *Quinoa risotto with rocket and parmesan* OR *Sweet potato cakes and baked tomatoes with rocket salad*
- Small mixed green salad
- 2 dried figs and six almonds

THROUGHOUT THE DAY

Snack mid-morning/afternoon (from the snack list)

- Daily relaxation 20 minutes

Weeks three and four

Congratulations! You have completed the first two weeks of the program. Reward yourself with a facial, a massage, a scrub or some other beauty treatment. And to stay motivated, remember that the one-month program will not only trigger a major turnaround in how your skin looks and feels but will also enhance your overall health and beauty! The real 'fountain of youth' is a healthy diet and life-style.

Your outer beauty really glows when you are healthy internally — physically, mentally and spiritually. So for the next two weeks, each morning practise deep breathing for radiant skin. Sit in a comfortable position. Open your chest by pulling your shoulder blades together. Let your chest expand and rise as you inhale slowly through your nose, and let it fall naturally as you exhale through your mouth. Do this for a few minutes every morning to give your skin a radiant glow for the day.

Remember to keep drinking at least 8 glasses of water per day (at least 1200ml). By keeping a bottle of purified, natural mineral or spring water with you throughout the day, you'll know how much you're actually drinking.

DAY 15: MONDAY

BREAKFAST

- *Natural Bircher muesli*
- Few slices of rockmelon
- Green tea/herbal tea
- Skin supplements

LUNCH

- *Roasted capsicum, tomato and chickpea salad*
- Slice of whole grain rye bread
- Skin supplements

DINNER

- *Poached seafood in lime and coconut dressing*
- $^1/_2$ cup brown rice
- Rocket and avocado salad

THROUGHOUT THE DAY

- Snack mid-morning/afternoon (from snack list)
- Some form of aerobic exercise or weight training
- Daily relaxation 20 minutes

> Hit the sack early — there's a reason it's called beauty sleep. Growth hormone and anti-ageing hormones like melatonin are produced in greater amounts at night. When we skimp on sleep, we don't allow our bodies to make these hormones in the quantities we need. This week aim for eight hours' sleep per night.

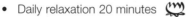

DAY 16: TUESDAY

BREAKFAST

- $^3/_4$ cup of low-fat natural yoghurt with fresh fruit (choose one or mix in rock-melon, honeydew, berries, peaches, plums or pears). Sprinkle with sliced almonds or walnuts and drizzle with a little raw honey to sweeten if desired. Add two tablespoons of freshly ground flax seeds.
- Skin supplements

LUNCH

- *Chickpea and broccoli salad with flaxseed–tahini dressing*
- Organic dried apricots with half a dozen raw almonds or walnuts
- Skin supplements

DINNER

- *Nut-crusted tuna* (or salmon)
- Steamed greens with olive oil and lemon juice
- Mixed salad with dark leafy greens, tomatoes, grated carrots, capsicums, chopped parsley. Dress with *ginger miso dressing*.

THROUGHOUT THE DAY

- Snack mid-morning/afternoon (from snack list)
- Some form of aerobic exercise or weight training ♡
- Daily relaxation 20 minutes

DAY 17: WEDNESDAY

BREAKFAST

- *Coconut berry smoothie*
- Green tea/herbal tea
- Skin supplements

LUNCH

- *Chicken salad Niçoise style*
- Low-GI fruit such as a pear, an apple or a peach
- Skin supplements

DINNER

- Grilled fish of choice from list, seasoned with fresh garlic, olive oil and freshly ground pepper
- Steamed mixed vegetables (broccoli, cauliflower, spinach, asparagus) tossed with virgin olive oil, lemon juice and garlic
- *Baked peaches with ricotta*

THROUGHOUT THE DAY

- Snack mid-morning/afternoon (from snack list)
- Some form of aerobic exercise or weight training ♡
- Daily relaxation 20 minutes

DAY 18: THURSDAY

BREAKFAST

- *Cavewoman muesli* served with fruit such as grated apple or berries. Add almond milk, soymilk, coconut cream/milk.
- Green tea/herbal tea
- Skin supplements

LUNCH

- Grilled salmon (can use canned salmon, just drain off liquid the way you do with tuna) and toss with cos lettuce, chopped celery, fresh coriander, small Spanish onion. Dress with olive oil and fresh lemon juice. One piece wholegrain rye bread.
- 2 dried figs and half a dozen almonds
- Skin supplements

DINNER

- Wholegrain/rice pasta with tomato vegetable sauce
- Small tossed green salad with avocado and walnuts
- Slices of apple with *almond cream*

THROUGHOUT THE DAY

- Snack mid-morning/afternoon (from snack list)
- Some form of aerobic exercise or weight training
- Daily relaxation 20 minutes

DAY 19: FRIDAY

BREAKFAST

- Organic figs covered with thick Greek yoghurt or organic yoghurt. Sprinkle with crushed walnuts, almonds, pecans or macadamia nuts.
- Green tea/herbal tea
- Skin supplements

LUNCH

- *Edamame salad with herbs*
- Small apple or pear
- Skin supplements

DINNER

- *Grilled miso salmon*
- *Broccoli stir-fry*
- $1/2$ cup brown rice
- *Spicy fruit compote*

THROUGHOUT THE DAY

- Snack mid-morning/afternoon (from snack list)
- Some form of aerobic exercise or weight training ♡ 🏋
- Daily relaxation 20 minutes 🧘

DAY 20: SATURDAY

BREAKFAST

- Vegetable and herb omelette made with 2 eggs and 1 cup sautéed vegetables in olive oil and served with freshly chopped herbs of choice
- Skin supplements 💊

LUNCH

- *Beetroot and green salad* with hard-boiled egg
- 1 apple or pear and 4 raw macadamia nuts
- Skin supplements 💊

DINNER

- *Pumpkin seed-crusted snapper*
- Mixed green salad with *tomato basil dressing*
- *Grilled fresh figs with macadamia nuts and ricotta*

THROUGHOUT THE DAY

- Snack mid-morning/afternoon (from snack list)
- Some form of aerobic exercise or weight training ♡ 🏋
- Daily relaxation 20 minutes 🧘

DAY 21: SUNDAY

BREAKFAST

- Scrambled eggs with fresh herbs and mushrooms, 1 slice wholegrain rye or gluten-free toast
- Tomato juice
- Skin supplements 💊

LUNCH

- *Lentil, goat's cheese and beetroot salad*
- Low-GI fruit and natural yoghurt
- Skin supplements

DINNER

- Grilled free-range chicken with *avocado salsa*
- Salad of dark-green leafy lettuces, tomatoes, mushrooms, fresh herbs, crumbled goat's cheese, slices of pears, chopped walnuts, and drizzled with extra-virgin olive oil, balsamic vinegar and lemon juice
- $1/2$ cup brown rice (for those who crave more carbs)

THROUGHOUT THE DAY

- Snack mid-morning/afternoon (from snack list)
- Daily relaxation 20 minutes

> Any woman can be beautiful. When asked to comment on the subject of beauty, actress Audrey Hepburn offered the following advice. 'For attractive lips, speak words of kindness. For lovely eyes, seek out the good in people. For a slim figure, share your food with the hungry. For poise, walk with the knowledge you'll never have to walk alone.'

DAY 22: MONDAY

BREAKFAST

- Mixed berry fruit salad (combine half-cup each strawberries, raspberries, and blueberries). Mix with juice of $1/4$ lemon and low-fat natural yoghurt and sprinkle with sliced almonds and shredded coconut.
- Green tea/herbal tea
- Skin supplements

LUNCH

- Chicken salad with skinless chicken breast, lettuce, cucumbers, avocado, walnuts, and dressed with lemon juice and olive oil
- 1 apple or a pear
- Skin supplements

DINNER

- *Barramundi with lime, ginger and shiitake mushrooms*
- Steamed asparagus and string beans
- Small tossed green salad
- *Peaches with toasted macadamia nuts and almond cream*

THROUGHOUT THE DAY

- Snack mid-morning/afternoon (from snack list)
- Some form of aerobic exercise or weight training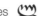
- Daily relaxation 20 minutes

> What you focus on expands. So this week focus on your inner beauty and self-esteem.

DAY 23: TUESDAY

BREAKFAST

- *Fruit and nut breakfast* served with coconut milk/cream, soy, almond or rice milk
- Green tea/herbal tea
- Skin supplements

LUNCH

- *Thai tofu salad*
- Handful of raw nuts and raisins
- Skin supplements

DINNER

- *Roasted ocean trout with pesto crust*
- Streamed vegetables of choice with fresh herbs, drizzled with olive oil and crushed pumpkin seeds or toasted pine nuts
- *Sweet potato mash*

THROUGHOUT THE DAY

- Snack mid-morning/afternoon (from snack list)
- Some form of aerobic exercise or weight training
- Daily relaxation 20 minutes

Have a massage! Not only does it feel fantastic but massage also stimulates circulation and skin renewal.

DAY 24: WEDNESDAY

BREAKFAST

- 2 eggs scrambled with one tablespoon olive oil, spinach or kale, onions and oregano
- Green tea/herbal tea
- Skin supplements

LUNCH

- *Rocket, walnut and apple salad*
- Organic dried apricots, handful sunflower seeds and raw nuts
- Skin supplements

DINNER

- *Steamed snapper with ginger and shallots*
- *Pawpaw and carrot salad*

THROUGHOUT THE DAY

- Snack mid-morning/afternoon (from snack list)
- Some form of aerobic exercise or weight training
- Daily relaxation 20 minutes

Mist your face. Dull, dry and dehydrated skin can magnify fine lines. For an instant dewy look, spritz on some Jurlique Rosewater spray.

DAY 25: THURSDAY

BREAKFAST

- *Whey protein blueberry shake*
- Skin supplements

LUNCH

- *Rocket salad with fennel and pine nuts*
- *Lentil and vegetable soup*
- Skin supplements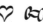

DINNER

- *Blue-eyed cod poached with saffron, fennel and tomato*
- Small tossed green salad with *flaxseed dressing*
- $1/2$ cup brown rice (optional)

THROUGHOUT THE DAY

- Snack mid-morning/afternoon (from snack list)
- Some form of aerobic exercise or weight training ♡ ⋈
- Daily relaxation 20 minutes ☕

DAY 26: FRIDAY

BREAKFAST

- Whole grapefruit cut in half. (Pink grapefruits make a tasty change and they're packed with the powerful phytonutrient lycopene also found in tomatoes, guava, and watermelon.)
- 1 poached free-range egg on whole rye toast
- Tomatoes grilled with olive oil and basil
- Skin supplements

LUNCH

- *Asparagus and lentil salad with tomato–lemon dressing*
- 1 apple or pear and 4 raw macadamia nuts
- Skin supplements

DINNER

- *Grilled red snapper with tomato salsa*
- *Asparagus with hazelnut gremolata*
- 2 slices rockmelon

THROUGHOUT THE DAY

- Snack mid-morning/afternoon (from snack list)
- Some form of aerobic exercise or weight training ♡ 🏋
- Daily relaxation 20 minutes 🔥

DAY 27: SATURDAY

BREAKFAST

- *Scrambled tofu* served with mushrooms, chives and fresh herbs
- 2 slices rockmelon
- Skin supplements 💊

LUNCH

- *Tuna, egg and bean salad*
- *Borscht*
- Skin supplements 💊

DINNER

- *Garden-style primavera with rice noodles*
- Tossed salad with a dressing of olive oil, red wine vinegar and a little fresh garlic
- Sliced apples and half a dozen almonds

THROUGHOUT THE DAY

- Snack mid-morning/afternoon (from snack list)
- Some form of aerobic exercise or weight training ♡ 🏋
- Daily relaxation 20 minutes 🔥

> Live in love. When you're in love, you glow. But you don't need to wait
> around for Cupid's arrow! You can get the same results by simply evoking a
> memory of love or even your favourite pet.

DAY 28: SUNDAY

BREAKFAST

- Half a grapefruit
- 1 soft-boiled egg on wholegrain rye bread

- 1 grilled tomato drizzled with olive oil and chopped herbs
- Green tea/herbal tea
- Skin supplements

LUNCH

- Avocado salad with ¹/₂ small avocado, lime juice, cucumbers, spring greens, tomatoes and shallots with 1 tablespoon flaxseed oil
- Grilled free-range chicken breast
- Skin supplements

DINNER

- Grilled fresh fish of your choice, brushed with olive oil, freshly ground pepper and sea salt. Serve with freshly chopped herbs.
- Steamed artichokes
- Mixed green salad

THROUGHOUT THE DAY

- Snack mid-morning/afternoon (from snack list)
- Daily relaxation 20 minutes

DAY 29: MONDAY

BREAKFAST

- Sliced fresh fruit (choose one or mix in rockmelon, honeydew, berries, peaches, plums or pears) with goat's or sheep's milk or natural yoghurt. Sprinkle with sliced almonds or walnuts and drizzle with a little raw honey to sweeten if desired. Add two tablespoons of freshly ground flax seeds.
- Green tea/herbal tea
- Skin supplements

LUNCH

- Salad Niçoise made with tuna, olives, green beans, and tomatoes with Cos lettuce and *Tomato basil dressing*
- Skin supplements

DINNER

- Grilled blue-fin tuna with *Avocado salsa*
- Steamed spinach or kale drizzled with olive oil
- Small mixed green salad dressed with olive oil/balsamic vinegar and fresh herbs

THROUGHOUT THE DAY

- Snack mid-morning/afternoon (from snack list)
- Some form of aerobic exercise or weight training ♡ 🏋
- Daily relaxation 20 minutes 🔥

DAY 30: TUESDAY

BREAKFAST

- Mash half an avocado onto wholegrain or dark rye bread
- Small fruit salad with slivered almonds and natural yoghurt
- Green tea/herbal tea
- Skin supplements 💊

LUNCH

- Small can of sardines/salmon/tuna in olive oil
- *Chickpea and broccoli salad with flax seed–tahini dressing*
- Skin supplements 💊

DINNER

- *Spinach frittata with tomato salsa*
- Steamed vegetables of choice such as spinach, broccoli, green beans or artichokes with fresh herbs, drizzled with olive oil and crushed pumpkin seeds
- *Spicy fruit compote* with natural yoghurt

THROUGHOUT THE DAY

- Snack mid-morning/afternoon (from snack list)
- Some form of aerobic exercise or weight training ♡ 🏋
- Daily relaxation 20 minutes 🔥

Recommended supplement and food lists

Please don't feel overwhelmed by all the different recipes and menu plans. The menu plan for the 30-day program is merely a guideline and is certainly not meant as a strict rule for what you must eat on any given day. The following lists give you scope to design your own meals if you wish. Feel free to be as creative as you like with the lists; just remember to stick to the foods outlined here.

Beauty-boosting supplements
To take on an empty stomach:

- L-Carnitine or Aceyl L-Carnitine — 500mg twice daily (on an empty stomach)
- Probiotics — ¹/₂ teaspoon twice daily on an empty stomach (away from food)

To take with breakfast:

- High-potency multi-vitamin and mineral × 1
- Vitamin C — 1000mg (1 gram)
- Alpha-lipoic acid — 50mg
- Coenzyme Q10 (COQ10) — 30mg
- EPA/DHA — 1000mg
- Grapeseed extract or pcynogenol — 30–100mg
- MSM — 1000mg

(In the winter months take 1 teaspoon of cod liver oil per day)

To take with lunch or dinner:

- Vitamin C — 1000mg (one gram)
- Alpha-lipoic acid — 50mg

- Coenzyme Q10 (COQ10) — 30mg
- EPA/DHA — 1000mg
- MSM — 1000mg
- Selenium — 25 micrograms take as selenomethione (organic form of selenium)

See the Resources section for further details about supplement sources.

❗ Always consult your doctor before taking any supplements, especially if you have a pre-existing medical condition or are pregnant or are on any medication.

Recommended vegetables

- Artichokes
- Asparagus
- Beans (green, Italian)
- Bean sprouts
- Beet greens
- Beetroot
- Bok choy
- Broccoli
- Brussels sprouts
- Capsicums (green, red, yellow and orange)
- Cabbage (green and red)
- Carrots
- Cauliflower
- Celery
- Cucumber
- Daikon§

- Dandelion greens
- Eggplant (Aubergine)
- Endive
- Escarole (broadleaf endive)
- Fennel
- Garlic
- Ginger (fresh)
- Kale
- Kohlrabi
- Lettuce (such as Cos and other dark leafy ones)
- Mushrooms
- Onions
- Parsley
- Pumpkin
- Radicchio
- Radishes

- Rocket
- Spinach
- Summer squash
- Tomatoes
- Turnips
- Watercress
- Zucchini

Daikon is a white radish. It can be grated fresh or steamed. It's used a lot in Japan and is believed to assist with digestion and the metabolism of fats.

Recommended fruits

- Apples
- Apricots
- Avocado
- Bananas
- Berries (blackberries, blueberries, raspberries, strawberries)
- Cherries
- Citrus fruits (lemons, oranges, mandarins)
- Figs
- Grapefruit
- Grapes
- Guava
- Honeydew melon
- Kiwifruit
- Mango
- Pawpaw
- Peaches
- Pears
- Plums
- Pomegranates
- Rhubarb
- Rockmelon

Recommended fish and seafood

- Barramundi
- Blue and Spanish mackerel
- Blue-eyed cod
- Gemfish
- Green-lipped NZ mussels
- Ocean trout
- Pacific herring
- Salmon
- Sardines
- Scallops
- Sea or Queensland mullet
- Snapper
- Tailor
- Tuna (Southern blue fin)

- Salmon (King and Atlantic) — wild where possible; canned is a great option because it's wild

Recommended poultry

- Free-range/organic chicken
- Free range organic eggs
- Free-range/organic turkey

Recommended legumes and grains

- Amaranth
- Barley (whole for soups)
- Beans (including black, chickpeas, lentils, lima, navy, pinto and soy)
- Brown rice
- Oatmeal (old-fashioned, coarse-ground, not instant)
- Quinoa

Recommended nuts and seeds

- Almonds
- Brazil nuts
- Cashews
- Chestnuts
- Flaxseeds
- Hazelnuts
- Macadamia nuts
- Pecans
- Pine nuts
- Pistachios (unsalted)
- Pumpkin seeds
- Sesame seeds (white and black)
- Sunflower seeds
- Walnuts

Recommended sources of whole soy

- Miso
- Soy milk/soy yoghurt
- Tempeh
- Tofu

Be sure that where possible you purchase organic soy products to ensure that they are not from GM soybeans.

Recommended dairy

- Low-fat yoghurt and regular plain yoghurt (organic where possible) without added sugar
- Goat's milk/sheep's milk yoghurt (organic where possible)
- Greek/Bulgarian feta cheese (from sheep's or goat's milk)
- Kefir
- Low-fat ricotta cheese

Recommended canned goods

- Alaskan (wild) salmon packed in water
- Chicken broth, no salt, no MSG or other additives
- Chickpeas (organic)
- Mackerel
- Olives
- Sardines packed in olive oil
- Tuna packed in water

Recommended salad and cooking oils

- Cold-pressed extra-virgin coconut oil
- Extra-virgin olive oil
- Flaxseed oil — organic, cold-pressed (**it must never be heated**)
- Macadamia nut oil—organic, cold-pressed
- Mustard seed oil (cold pressed)
- Walnut oil — cold pressed (**it must never be heated**)

Recommended condiments

- Celtic sea salt
- Mustards (grain and smooth — without honey)
- Natural almond and soy nut butters
- Sesame tahini
- Tamari (wheat-free soy sauce)

Recommended beverages

- Green tea (hot or iced)
- Herbal teas
- Pomegranate juice
- Spring water, filtered or natural mineral water
- Teechino herbal coffees (See Resources)
- Unsweetened cranberry juice

Recommended herbs

- Basil
- Bay leaf
- Dill
- Mint
- Oregano
- Rosemary
- Sage
- Tarragon
- Thyme

Recommended spices

- Cinnamon
- Coriander
- Cumin
- Ginger
- Paprika
- Turmeric

Congratulations! You have finished the one-month program and are on the path to a lifetime of health and fabulous skin. You should be feeling fantastic and sparkling with vitality, and your face should look fresh and rejuvenated. The best news is that you should now be motivated to continue eating the Gorgeous Skin way as the healthy glow of gorgeous skin reflects a healthy body. You should also feel empowered as you now have the tools to make healthy lifestyle choices that will affect how you look and feel inside and out.

9

Gorgeous Skin for a Special Occasion

Reasons to Glow

There are many times when we want to look our best for a special occasion or event. It may be your wedding or your son's or daughter's wedding. Or perhaps you want to look your best at a reunion, family gathering or for a graduation or award ceremony. There are so many occasions when we might want to put our best face forward. How you look on your special day will help your confidence and even your enjoyment of the day. You'll want to look as picture perfect as possible. A stunning outfit and excellent grooming are essential, but just as important is having radiantly beautiful skin. Unfortunately no amount of makeup on your special day can conceal a dull, sallow, stressed-out complexion, no matter how many facials, micro-dermabrasion or other beauty treatments you have had. Make sure you plan time to look after your inner health and beauty. Remember, your skin is a direct reflection of your diet and lifestyle, so eating well and really healthily in the weeks leading up to your wedding or special occasion will give you a radiant glow that no ordinary skincare or makeup can!

There are very few quick fixes you can make just before your big day, but you can reap huge rewards from medium- to long-term changes to your diet and lifestyle. Remember: when you look at your skin you're looking at the result of your last thirty-day skin renewal cycle. So the biggest impact you can have on getting gorgeous skin for your wedding day is to make changes to your diet and lifestyle as early on as you can! For radiant, picture-perfect skin on your special day, you've got to start eating well at least one month, or ideally two months, before the big occasion.

Feed your face

So many women eat with weight reduction in mind, not their skin or beauty, especially before their wedding. They cut kilojoules, fat and other essential nutrients like nobody's business. But this is one of the worst things you can possibly do, as your skin cells need a nutrient-rich, highly oxygenated blood supply and plenty of mineral building blocks to look their absolute best, plus lots of good fats to give your skin a hydrated, soft and supple look. The freshest fruit and vegetables, lean protein from cold-water fish and free-range poultry, complex carbohydrates (low GI and non-starchy) and good fats from nuts and olive oil are the best cosmetics around and they will get you glowing in no time.

The goal of the bride-to-be Gorgeous Skin plan is to maximise nutrition to include foods packed with antioxidants, vitamins, minerals, phytonutrients and good fats. Just as important are the foods you should give up for the sake of your skin. The aim is to maximise great nutrition and minimise poor food choices and empty kilojoules. Here are some of the simple rules.

Forget going low fat!

You can't cut out fat and expect gorgeous, radiant skin for your wedding day. Your skin needs good fats to give you a rosy glow and a dewy, well-hydrated complexion. If you cut out fats for the sake of fitting into your beautiful dress, your skin will look lacklustre, dry and dehydrated. Nor can you cut kilojoules to nothing and expect your skin to look radiantly beautiful. Your skin needs good fats. Make sure you are having at least two tablespoons of fats such as olive oil or flax seed oil every day.

! If you're getting fewer than 20 grams of fat a day (roughly 2 tablespoons of oil), your skin may not be able to lubricate itself and your body may not absorb enough vitamin A, which your skin needs to look its absolute best.

Don't cut kilojoules dramatically

Cut kilojoules dramatically and you'll find yourself in short supply of protein, essential fats, vitamins and minerals, all at the expense of your skin (not to mention your general health). Your skin cells need a nutrient-rich, highly oxygenated blood supply and plenty of minerals, as well as other nutrients like fats and protein, to look their absolute best. So even if you're trying to lose a few kilos, if you follow the eating plan you will lose weight, gradually and healthily. Don't forget to exercise, either … this way you'll really boost your metabolism plus beat stress.

Cut out the refined carbohydrates and sugar

If you do only one thing, cut out *all* forms of sugar and refined carbohydrates! Sugar robs your cells of vital nutrients, generates free radicals, causes cross-linking of collagen, and results in youth-stealing spikes of insulin from high levels of blood sugar. It can also aggravate all forms of acne.

Be careful though: sugar sneaks into almost everything we eat, and not just the obvious cakes, biscuits and soft drinks. In fact, it's hidden in virtually all packaged and processed foods. Check all labels for sugar listed as not only sugar but also dextrose, high fructose corn syrup, sucrose, rice syrup and table sugar.

All refined carbohydrates break down in your body to sugar, too. These in turn will cause your blood sugar levels to rise sky high. So for your goal of radiantly beautiful skin, cut out all refined carbohydrates such as cakes, biscuits, pastries, bagels, donuts, pretzels, corn chips, sweets, white and milk chocolate, pizza and junk food. Ditto for white pasta, which most people think of as a healthy meal (it's really just a simple sugar). If you do indulge, never eat sugars on an empty stomach. For example, a bagel and a coffee for breakfast is a pure sugar rush! There's no protein and good

 TIP

Can't bear the thought of giving up bread? Try whole-grain rye bread, or have sushi for lunch instead of sandwiches.

fats to hold back the great surge of sugar you'll get and you'll be hungry again in a few hours and possibly irritable too. It will also do absolutely nothing to keep a gorgeous waistline for your wedding. And it certainly won't contribute towards your wedding day glow either! Refined carbohydrates can also make you retain water and cause bloating, which is something you especially want to avoid just before your wedding.

Eliminate empty kilojoules

Avoid empty kilojoules, including all low-joule and no-joule food and drinks such as Diet Coke and Pepsi, non-fat/full-of-sugar foods, and non-fat fruit yoghurts, as they're loaded with sugar but devoid of nutrients.

Say goodbye to processed foods

Read the labels and avoid all additives, MSG, preservatives, artificial colours and anything that you can't pronounce. You want optimum nutrition to look as gorgeous as possible and most processed foods contain so few nutrients that you might as well be eating the cardboard box!

Forgo all fried

Skip all hot chips, deep-fried spring rolls and all your favourite comfort junk food. It will seriously undo all your good work. The fats in fried food are trans fats: they increase inflammation and free radical damage, and can displace all the good fats in your cell membranes, making it more difficult for nutrients to pass into your cells — including your skin cells. (Miss out on the margarine, too — it's a major trans fat trap.)

Go low GI

Fill up on fibre found in non-starchy, low-GI vegetables, fruits, whole grains such as brown rice and legumes. Flip to the charts in Chapter 2 to see the GI levels of various foods.

Relax

All the frenzied wedding planning and organising can make your body pump out lots of stress hormones, which is bad news for your skin. Under stress your body redirects critical nutrients from your skin to your vital organs, such as your heart, brain and lungs, and over time this process deprives your skin of oxygen and nourishment, resulting in less-than-gorgeous skin. Extended periods of stress (like the months of preparations for your wedding) also affect your metabolic functions by slowing down the renewal of your skin cells, leading to dull, grey skin.

When you're under pressure, you also tend to tighten your muscles, and this restricts blood flow to your skin cells. At the same time, it can slow down the lymphatic drainage into and out of every organ, so that your cells can't defend themselves from infection. You may notice you have dull, sallow skin that is prone to spots, strange bumps and allergic reactions and chapped lips that are susceptible to sores. This is because the stress response also amplifies free radical production! So remember to relax as often as possible. You can keep your stress levels in check by doing some form of regular relaxation. Exercise will also boost circulation and help you feel calm and centred over the months before the wedding.

When you're relaxed your superficial circulation increases, your hormone output improves, especially the hormones that control healing and cell replication, and you benefit from more endorphins, the hormones that create the 'feel-good' factor. Yoga, meditation, qi gong and tai chi are some of the most powerful ways to create beautiful skin from within. Try to do something calming and relaxing every day for the month leading up to your wedding.

Move

Try any exercise you enjoy — such as dancing, yoga, Pilates, cycling, or a brisk walk — to relieve pre-wedding stress as often as you can. It will get your heart pumping, which in turn increases oxygen and nutrients to your skin's surface, and will help you release feel-good endorphins! Exercise at least four times a week. Also if you want to shed a few extra kilos before your wedding or special event, this will boost the effects of a healthy diet. See the section on 'Losing it' later in the chapter.

Sleep well

Don't skimp on sleep before your wedding. Sleep replenishes, rejuvenates and restores. A chronic lack of sleep will take its toll on your complexion. Your skin's rate of cell renewal (a function essential for fresh, young-looking skin) is at its highest when we sleep. It is essential that you schedule at least seven to eight hours of deep, restful sleep per night.

Get as much sleep as possible the night before your big day. But not so much that you're left with pillow creases on your face and puffy eyes!

Hydrate

At least one month before your big occasion (if you're not doing it already) you should be drinking at least 1.5 to 2 litres of water a day. Water hydrates your skin cells and will leave your skin looking smoother and visibly younger. It's also vital for diluting and expelling toxins as well as helping to prevent blemishes.

Avoid alcohol

 TIP
Instead of a traditional hens' night, why not go with your bridesmaids or girlfriends for a weekend of spa treatments or head to a health resort. You'll emerge restored, rejuvenated and feeling fantastic. (See Resources.)

Although it's one of the most tempting times to indulge in a drink or two, alcohol really does sap your skin's moisture and deplete its levels of nutrients such as the stress-busting and skin-beautifying B vitamins. The occasional glass of red wine is OK; and if you do indulge, follow with a large glass of water. Of course your hens' night is an exception, but make sure you follow each drink with a large glass of water and end the night with extra antioxidants!

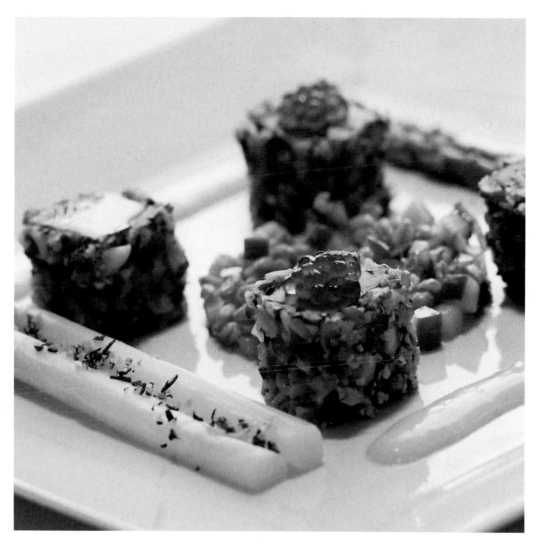

Turn tuna's good fats and oils into glowing skin with the scrumptious **Nut crusted tuna** rolled in hazelnut gremolata and served with asparagus.

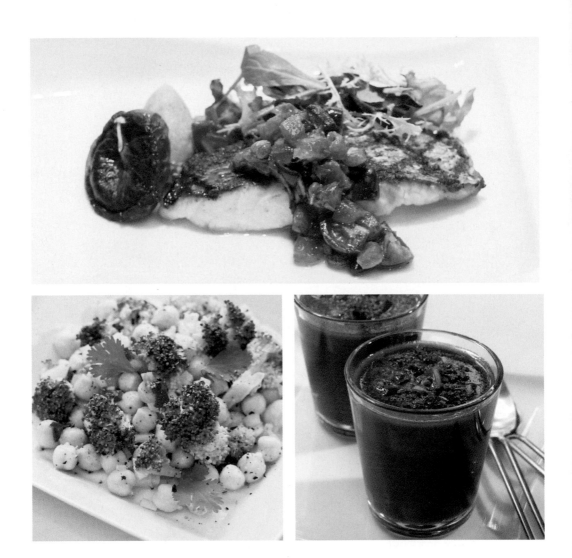

Boost your lycopene levels with tasty **Gazpacho**, get lots of fibre with the appetizing **Chickpea and broccoli salad**, and get more beauty boosting fish oils with the juicy **Grilled red snapper** topped with tomato salsa.

Detoxify to get glowing wedding-day skin

Flip to the chapter on detoxification (Chapter Seven) for an added beauty boost. Be warned, though: *don't* detoxify directly before the big day, otherwise you'll feel and look terrible and will have all the accompanying unpleasant side-effects, including bad breath and skin eruptions! Any radical changes to your diet can cause your skin to break out. This won't last forever, but it's certainly not something you want just before your wedding. If you can, do the detox before you start this plan, but make sure you detox at least one month (two months would be ideal) before your wedding day. Then you can follow the Gorgeous Skin plan for brides as faithfully as possible up until your big day.

Bride-to-be Gorgeous Skin plan

Remember your skin cells have a rapid turnover and are replaced on average every month. If you can, start your Gorgeous Skin plan earlier than 28 days beforehand — two months if possible.

Time is of the essence, and the last thing you need is to be overwhelmed with huge amounts of information and a complicated daily plan, so you'll find here a list of menu samples for breakfast, lunch and dinner, plus a snack list. You'll also find a list of supplements to take twice daily. Each of the meal suggestions is loaded with antioxidants and packed with healthy protein, carbohydrates and fat for gorgeous skin.

There are a few key rules you need to remember. When thinking of any meal you want to include the following three things:

- lean protein
- good fats
- good carbohydrates (low GI, non-starchy).

It's a simple as ABC—but we'll call it good PFC (protein, fat and carbs) instead! For protein you could choose a piece of fish (grilled, steamed or poached); for fats and carbohydrates, a salad with Cos lettuce, avocado and capsicum, with a dressing of olive oil and balsamic vinegar or lemon juice, and a slice of wholegrain rye bread. This meal includes your good fats (avocado and olive oil) and good carbs (dark rye bread and vegies). This way you'll balance out your blood sugar and energy levels, will get all your essential nutrients and will feel full and satisfied for longer.

There are ten selections each for breakfast, lunch and dinner. Keep in mind that these are only suggestions, so feel free to mix and match and to swap lunch meals with dinner. Try to vary your diet as much as possible and remember to include the good fats, carbs and lean protein with every meal. You'll get the hang of it after a while. If you do slip up, just get back on track by following the plan again. Or just think fruits, vegetables, fish, olive oil and some raw nuts! All of these foods help create beauty from within.

The dietary guidelines are simple:

- Stick to the PFCs (lean protein, good fats from olive oil or raw unsalted nuts and good carbs for each meal).
- Eat plenty of fresh fruit and vegetables, especially deep and vibrantly coloured ones, like blueberries and spinach.
- Go whole grain.
- Include good fats such as olive oil, raw nuts, and avocado daily.
- Drink 6 to 8 glasses of water per day.
- Up your intake of deep-sea fish. It contains the healthiest skin fats.
- To keep your blood sugar levels stable don't go longer than four hours without eating.
- Take the supplements twice a day where possible. This will boost the effects of your Gorgeous Skin plan.
- Avoid all the skin baddies (cut out the whites: sugar, white bread, refined pasta, white rice and table salt).
- Start each day with a herbal tea, deep breathing, stretching, yoga, meditation or a walk. It will give you a sense of calm so you can achieve all the things you need to get done.

Breakfast

Breakfast is an absolute must, to balance out your blood sugar levels and give you energy to start the day. If time is an issue, add some fruit to natural yoghurt, and sprinkle with chopped nuts such as walnuts or almonds. Or whiz up a *whey protein blueberry shake*. Otherwise, choose from the following (italics indicate that a recipe can be found in Chapter 10).

- *Natural Bircher muesli* or *Cavewoman muesli*.
- Poached egg on wholegrain rye toast, grilled tomato, half a grape-fruit.
- 3/4 cup yogurt (plain, organic) with fruit such as blueberries, topped with 1 tablespoon slivered almonds and 2 tablespoon freshly ground flax seeds
- 1/2 cup oatmeal (not the instant kind) with soymilk, rice milk or coconut cream/milk and topped with chopped walnuts, blueberries and grated apple
- Eggwhite omelette, 1 serving fruit.
- Smoothie with whey protein powder, berries, soy or rice milk.
- *Scrambled tofu*, a few slices of rockmelon.
- Half a punnet of blueberries, 1/2 cup organic plain yoghurt and 2 teaspoons crushed hazelnuts or almonds topped with shredded coconut.
- Scrambled eggs with spinach, mushrooms and chopped herbs.
- Fresh fruit salad topped with natural yoghurt and crushed raw nuts and freshly ground flax seed.

Lunch

Keep in mind that the lunch and dinner meals are just suggestions: feel free to mix and match any of the proteins and vegetables, as long as they are on the approved food item list. Don't forget the PFCs rule, either (protein, fat and carbs with every meal) — add some delicious protein sources to your salad, such as grilled free-range chicken, fish (salmon/sardines/mackerel packed in water or olive oil), eggs, tofu or prawns. Crumbled feta, avocado, toasted pine nuts and walnuts make tasty and nutritious additions. Try to avoid commercial salad dressing if possible. Make your own and take it with you: a few teaspoons of extra-virgin olive oil, balsamic vinegar or fresh lemon juice, and chopped herbs.

- Can of salmon, salad of rocket, tomatoes, olives, avocado, capsicums, olive oil and balsamic dressing, piece wholegrain rye/gluten-free bread.
- Grilled chicken breast, tossed green salad, piece fruit.
- *Greek salad* with tuna, handful of almonds, piece of fruit.
- *Avocado and rocket salad*, tin of sardines/mackerel in olive oil, slice of wholegrain rye bread.
- *Lentil and vegetable soup*, piece of wholegrain rye bread.
- *Chickpea and broccoli salad with flax seed–tahini dressing*, handful of raisins and raw nuts.
- *Thai tofu salad*, handful of raisins and raw nuts.
- *Chicken salad Niçoise style*, slice of wholegrain rye or pumpernickel bread.
- *Asparagus and lentil salad with tomato-lemon dressing*, 1–2 slices of gluten-free bread or corn/rice crispbread.

Dinner

Vegies, vegies and more vegies! Your fish, chicken and vegetables should be steamed, grilled, poached or roasted rather than fried or sautéed. If you like to cook, indulge your creativity with fresh fish, vegetables and herbs. If you're eating out, steer friends to a restaurant where you can find healthy choices such as fish and salads.

- Grilled snapper with herbs, olive oil and lemon, *Spinach and egg salad with sprouts, mushrooms and radishes.*

- Grilled free-range chicken with *Avocado salsa* and mixed green salad.
- Grilled tuna brushed with olive oil and garlic, steamed broccoli, spinach and cauliflower, small mixed green salad.
- Wholegrain/corn/rice pasta with vegetable and tomato sauce, mixed salad.
- Grilled fish of choice, *Sweet potato mash*, rocket and Parmesan salad.
- *Borscht*, mixed green salad with avocado and pine nuts.
- Grilled salmon over rocket, sliced tomatoes, thick-sliced onions and black olives, $1/2$ cup brown rice.
- Grilled blue-fin tuna with *Salsa*, steamed spinach or kale drizzled with olive oil; small mixed green salad with avocado.
- Braised tofu with shiitake mushrooms and brown rice, mixed green salad.
- *Grilled miso salmon*, roast sweet potatoes, mixed green salad.

Snacks

Don't go hungry! Always pack some healthy snacks for when you get the munchies.

- Corn or rice crispbreads spread with hummus or with *Creamy hummus dip*.
- Unsalted seeds and raw nuts (two tablespoons).
- Soy yoghurt (add a few raw nuts or fruit).
- Tamari roasted almonds (a few tablespoons).
- *Almond, coconut and banana power muffins*.
- Raw vegetable sticks dipped in hummus.
- *Whey protein berry shake*.
- Apple slices dipped in almond butter.
- Homemade trail mix of almonds, pistachios, pumpkin seeds, macadamias, sunflower seeds, shredded coconut and organic raisins (a few tablespoons).

- Edamame (whole green soybeans boiled in their skins for ten minutes in salty water).

Drinks

- Water (filtered, spring or mineral)
- Herbal teas
- Green or black tea
- Sparkling mineral water with a splash of cranberry or grape juice
- Freshly squeezed fruit and vegetable juices like carrot, celery, apple, pear, ginger, pineapple
- Coffee substitutes such as Teeccino herbal coffees

Supplements

To take with breakfast:

- High-potency multi-vitamin and mineral × 1
- Vitamin C — 1000mg (1 gram)
- Alpha-lipoic acid — 50mg
- Coenzyme Q10 (COQ10) — 30mg
- EPA/DHA — 1000mg

To take with lunch or dinner:

- Vitamin C — 1000mg (1 gram)
- Alpha-lipoic acid — 50mg
- Coenzyme Q10 (COQ10) — 30mg
- EPA/DHA — 1000mg

! Always consult your doctor before taking any supplements, especially if you have a pre-existing medical condition or are pregnant or are taking any medication.

The daily do-gooders

Perfect protein: Deep-sea fish like salmon, tuna, mackerel and other fish filled with great skin fats, such as sardines. Free-range turkey and chicken, organic free-range cuts of lean meats, organic eggs, whey protein, whole unprocessed soy products, and yoghurt (organic where possible).

Good carbs: Green leafy vegetables such as spinach, Cos lettuce, broccoli, asparagus, beans, tomatoes, mushrooms, sweet potatoes, capsicums, cauliflower, carrots, cherries, blueberries, plums, kiwi fruit, peaches, pears, apples, rockmelon, whole oats, rye and other 'real' wholegrain breads, brown rice, quinoa, barley, chickpeas, lentils, millet, buckwheat and wild rice.

Fabulous fats: Good fats include virgin cold-pressed olive and coconut oil, fresh raw nuts such as almonds, hazelnuts, pecans, macadamias and walnuts, seeds like sunflower and pumpkin, olives, avocadoes, macadamia, cold-pressed flaxseed oil, flax seeds.

Add excitement: Toasted sesame seeds, crushed pumpkin seeds, fresh and dried herbs such as basil, coriander, dill and parsley, spices, ginger, crushed garlic and tamari (wheat-free soy sauce).

 TIP

Remember to take a moment to de-stress during your wedding week. Try not to get so swept up in the occasion that you lose sight of what's going on. Delegate what you can and let others do the worrying! Have a massage. Take a bath. Go for a long morning run; whatever it takes to calm you down and help you unwind.

Losing it

If you feel you need to shed a few unwanted kilos, set a real goal that you can achieve during wedding planning months without feeling stressed-out or pressured. Let's be realistic, though: it's not a good idea to try to lose a great deal of weight too close to your wedding date, or to set unrealistic fitness goals during a stressful time in your life. To lose weight healthily, set your sights on losing about one kilogram of weight a week — any more and you'll be losing not just your fat but your muscle as well.

Don't forget that a healthy diet and plenty of exercise will make you feel less tired and less stressed too. Whether you want to just tone up before the big day or lose a few kilos, follow the tips below.

Follow the PFCs rule

For every meal and snack include good protein, carbs and fat. When you eat foods with a low-glycaemic index (fruits, vegetables, beans) combined with protein (lean meats, seafood, soy) and fat (olive oil, fish oil, nuts), there is a long and slow build-up of blood sugar levels to sustain you over many hours and reduce the feeling of hunger.

Build muscles

Cardio alone won't do the trick. Add weight training three days a week. Toning muscles not only shapes your body but gets your metabolism going and helps you burn more fat. The more lean muscle you have, the faster your metabolism.

Aerobics

Not just the Jane Fonda kind, either! If possible do 30 to 60 minutes a day of some kind of aerobic activity, whether it be walking, jogging, elliptical training machine, swimming, dancing, or anything you can think of that gets your heart pumping. The trick is doing it almost every day. It will help you burn more kilojoules and by burning fat to its fullest potential, you can get in shape for your wedding day and stay in shape.

Breakfast

Never, ever skip breakfast. If you don't eat in the morning, your body thinks you're starving it, and will slow down your metabolism to a crawl to conserve. Eating the first meal of the day actually helps you to burn more kilojoules! Remember to eat protein with each meal too.

Bird-eaters beware

Always thought eating only a few bites will help you lose weight? Not so. Don't consume fewer than 5000 kilojoules a day, no matter what. Less than that, and your body can't support its own organ and muscle function; much less help you with other things, like thinking. In addition, just like skipping breakfast, your body believes you're starving it, and slows down to conserve, hanging on to every fat cell you ever had. So keep eating. It will actually help to keep you thinner and healthier in the long run.

Eat early

Food eaten earlier in the day generates more energy than food eaten later in the day. Your metabolic rate is actually higher earlier on in the day, which helps you to burn off kilojoules as energy, whereas these same kilojoules consumed at night can be easily stored as fat. So try to eat most of your daily kilojoules and nothing much after 6 to 7 p.m.

Walk

Along with your daily exercise, try to walk at least 10 to 30 minutes a day. This can actually be accomplished pretty easily — a short walk around the block after dinner, taking the stairs instead of the lift. This extra boost of activity can make a difference in the kilojoules you burn.

TIP

For a gorgeous sun-kissed glow, fake it! Most spas have a self-tanning treatment where they ensure you are suitably exfoliated, buffed and moisturised to avoid the streaky look. For best results, do a trial run a few months before your wedding. Or try an air-brushed or 'spray-on' tan. These last about a week, but make sure you try them out well before your wedding and find a colour that complements your skin tone. The active ingredient in these spray-on tans is dihydroxyacid (DHA), a safe, natural sugar derivative. Spray-on tans cover most blemishes and spider veins and will give you a sun-kissed look.

Active situations

Look for 'active situations' throughout your day. Park far from the shops so you have to walk more, use the stairs instead of lifts and escalators, get off a station earlier and walk the rest of the way, and other smaller activities to keep your body moving. Not only will this keep your body burning kilojoules at a maximum, you'll also notice a general increase in your energy level from all the activity, which is always great during stressed-out wedding planning!

Also you have to manage stress, because if it's your wedding you're preparing for it may be a time when you'll be the most stressed out of all. Weddings take so much planning and you will most likely spend over 100 hours on the phone, visiting suppliers, shopping, planning, and chasing after details! So the bride-to-be plan is designed to be as easy as possible.

There are so many special occasions when you want to look your absolute best — such as at your twenty-year school reunion, when you want to shine as the mother of the bride, at the start of a new romance or on a trip of a lifetime. You want results, and you want them fast. Diet is the quickest way to have a big impact on your skin's appearance as each and every one of your skin cells are fed by tiny capillaries that come from your blood — which means that they get their nourishment from what you eat and drink. Of course, you've still got to look after your skin externally too. Follow this plan as faithfully as possible and you'll start to see great results even in as little as a few days. And you'll feel fantastic as well.

The Recipes

Breakfast recipes

Soups/broth

Salads

Chicken recipe

Red meat

Noodle dish

Vegetable dishes

Dips and snacks

Desserts

Breakfast recipes

WHEY PROTEIN BLUEBERRY SHAKE

1–2 scoops (20–30 grams) micro-filtered whey protein powder or whey
    protein isolate powder (see Resources)
$1/2$ cup natural yoghurt OR $1/2$ cup organic soymilk OR $1/2$ cup organic
    rice milk
Handful of frozen or fresh organic berries
$1/2$ cup filtered water
2 ice cubes

Optional extras or variations:
1 tablespoon almonds
1 tablespoon sunflower seeds
1 organic egg
Frozen or fresh peaches other fruit of choice
1 organic banana
1 tablespoon flaxseed oil

Place all the ingredients into a blender and whiz vigorously until
combined.

COCONUT BERRY SMOOTHIE

200g natural yoghurt / organic goat's milk yoghurt OR 200g organic
    coconut milk
1 tablespoon extra-virgin coconut oil
$1/2$–1 cup of fresh or frozen fruit (berries, bananas, pineapple, etc.)
1 raw organic whole egg (optional)
1 tablespoon cold-pressed flaxseed oil
1 tablespoon raw unheated honey OR 1 tablespoon xylitol
1–2 scoops whey protein powder

Blend the ingredients in a high-speed blender.

NATURAL BIRCHER MUESLI

(Makes 4 servings)

$^3/_4$ cup unprocessed rolled oats
$^3/_4$ cup water (filtered or spring water)
2 tablespoons lemon juice
2 tablespoons plain yoghurt
2 green apples, unpeeled, cored, and grated
1–2 tablespoons raw or lightly toasted nuts such as almonds,
    walnuts or pecans

Soak rolled oats in the water overnight. In the morning add the remaining ingredients, sweetening to taste. Serve immediately with extra
yoghurt and freshly chopped fruit such as strawberries and pears.

CAVEWOMAN MUESLI

1 cup each:
Chopped raw almonds or almond meal
Chopped raw cashews
Hazelnut meal
Sunflower seeds
Shredded coconut
Brown rice puffs/flakes (optional)

Mix all ingredients in a large bowl. Spread thinly on a baking tray
and bake in a moderate oven for approximately 10 minutes (or until
the mixture turns golden). Remove from oven and allow to cool. Store
in an airtight container in the fridge. Serve with rice milk, almond
milk or coconut cream/milk and fruit (e.g. with stewed or grated
apple, berries, or sliced banana).

(Recipe courtesy of the Pro Health Clinic, Sydney)

FRUIT AND NUT BREAKFAST

2 portions of fresh fruit (e.g. strawberries, apples, etc.)
1 portion of stewed fruit (e.g. pears, peaches, etc.)
Generous handful of raw cashews
Generous handful of raw almonds
Sprinkle of sunflower seeds
Rice milk, almond milk or coconut milk/cream

Mix fresh fruit, stewed fruit, nuts and seeds in a cereal bowl. Add rice milk, almond milk or coconut milk/cream.

(Recipe courtesy of the Pro Health Clinic, Sydney)

ALMOND MILK

1 cup almonds
2 cups filtered water

Place almonds in blender and blend until they become a meal (usually about 60 seconds). Add water and blend for another 60 seconds. Pour mixture through a strainer into a container.

(Recipe courtesy of the Pro Health Clinic, Sydney)

PRAWN AND AVOCADO OMELETTE

(1 serving)

1 teaspoon olive oil
2 eggs
3 or 4 cooked prawns, chopped roughly
$1/4$ cup grated parmesan cheese
$1/4$ red ripe tomato, diced
$1/4$ ripe avocado, diced
1 tablespoon chopped fresh coriander (optional)
Sea salt & freshly ground black pepper

Prepare ingredients (prawns, cheese, tomato, avocado and coriander) before starting to cook. In a small bowl, toss tomato, avocado and coriander (if using). Season to taste with salt and pepper. Set aside. Beat the eggs in a small bowl just until the whites and yolks are combined, not long enough to become frothy. Over a medium–high heat, add the olive oil. Pour the eggs into the hot skillet, tilting and shaking the pan gently with one hand while stirring the eggs gently with a fork held flat with the other hand. When the eggs begin to firm up, add the prawns and cheese in a line along the centre third of the omelette. Immediately use a fork to fold one side then the other up over the centre filling, tilting the pan to help you 'roll' it into a loose cylinder. Cook another 10–30 seconds, depending on how brown you prefer the bottom (check for brownness by lifting a corner). Slide the omelette onto a warmed plate, top with tomato/avocado mixture and serve.

 TIP

If you are cooking for more than one person, make multiple 2-egg omelettes and keep the finished ones (without the topping) on warmed plates in an oven heated to 90 degrees Celsius until ready to serve.

SPINACH FRITTATA WITH TOMATO SALSA

(Makes 2 servings)

Frittata:
1 tablespoon extra-virgin olive oil
1 small sliced onion
2 cloves garlic, finely chopped or crushed
1 x 250g package frozen spinach, thawed and well drained, OR two bunches
   of steamed spinach
2 large organic or free-range eggs
3 egg whites
1/4 cup freshly grated parmesan

Salsa:
4 plum tomatoes, seeded and chopped
2 spring onions OR equivalent chives, minced
1 clove garlic, minced
2 tablespoons chopped fresh coriander
1 tablespoon fresh lime juice
1/4 teaspoon salt
1/8 teaspoon freshly ground black pepper

To make the frittata: Preheat the oven to 180 degrees Celsius. Heat the oil in a frypan over medium heat. Add the garlic and onion and cook, stirring for three minutes or until tender. Stir in the spinach. Reduce the heat to low. In a large bowl beat the eggs and egg whites until frothy. Pour the egg mixture over the spinach in the frypan. Cook for 5–7 minutes, until the egg mixture is cooked on the bottom and almost set on the top. Sprinkle lightly with the cheese. Bake in the oven until the eggs are set and the cheese has melted (5–10 minutes).

To make the salsa: In a large bowl, stir together the tomatoes, spring onions, garlic, coriander, lime juice, salt and pepper. Serve fresh, at room temperature, over the frittata.

SCRAMBLED TOFU #1

(Serves 4)

1 onion diced
2 stalks celery, finely diced
1–2 teaspoons olive oil
Turmeric to taste
450g firm or extra-firm tofu
Tamari (wheat-free soy sauce) to taste

Sauté turmeric for 1 minute. Add vegetables, starting with onion. Sauté 3–5 minutes. Crumble tofu and add to vegetables. Cook, covered, for 10–15 minutes, stirring occasionally.

SCRAMBLED TOFU #2

(Serves 4)

1 tablespoon olive oil or coconut oil
1/2 medium chopped green capsicum
1/2 medium red capsicum
6 mushrooms, chopped
450g firm tofu, drained and mashed with a fork

1 tablespoon mirin (Japanese rice wine)
1 tablespoon tamari
1 teaspoon dried or fresh basil
$^1/_2$ teaspoon granulated garlic
$^1/_2$ teaspoon curry powder
Freshly ground pepper to taste

Sauté onion, capsicums and mushrooms in oil for 3 minutes. Add tofu, mirin, tamari and herbs. Cook for 5 minutes, stirring frequently. Adjust seasonings to taste and sprinkle with black pepper.

Soups/broth

GAZPACHO

(Best if chilled for at least 2 hours before serving)

8 large ripe tomatoes
2 red capsicums
2 medium red onions
2 large cucumbers
$^1/_2$ cup red wine vinegar
$^1/_2$ cup olive oil
$1^1/_2$ cups tomato juice (canned)
1 tablespoon lemon juice (fresh)
1 teaspoon chopped coriander (fresh)
1 chilli (roughly chopped), fresh or dry
1 teaspoon cumin seed
1–2 cloves garlic
1 teaspoon oregano
Cracked black pepper and sea salt to taste
$^1/_4$ bunch spring onions or coriander leaves (for garnish, if desired)

Wash and prepare vegetables. Core and coarsely chop tomatoes. (Save the juice.) Core, seed and coarsely chop capsicums. Peel and coarsely chop onions. Peel, seed, and coarsely chop cucumbers. In a small bowl whisk together vinegar, olive oil, reserved tomato juice, canned tomato juice, lemon juice, garlic, herbs and spices.

In a blender or food processor (fitted with steel blade) purée vegetables in small batches, adding tomato juice mixture as needed to keep blade from clogging. (Do not purée completely; the gazpacho should retain some of its crunch.) Stir in salt and pepper to taste. Chill.

Ladle into chilled soup bowls or mugs and garnish with chopped spring onions or coriander leaves.

MISO VEGETABLE SOUP

(Makes 6 servings)

2 cups filtered water
2 cloves fresh garlic, minced or crushed
3–5 pieces of fresh peeled ginger (the size of a 10-cent coin)
200g tofu, cubed
2 teaspoons tamari or 1 tablespoon organic soy sauce
3 shiitake mushrooms, sliced
2 large dark-green leaves of spinach, bok choy or any other leafy vegetable
1^1/$_2$ tablespoons miso
1 spring onion, sliced
^{1}/$_4$ teaspoon toasted sesame oil (optional)
Sliced shallots for garnish

In a medium-sized saucepan, bring the water to a boil. While the water is heating, add the garlic, ginger, tofu, and tamari or soy sauce. When the water boils, lower the heat, cover the pot and simmer for 5 minutes. Add the mushrooms and spinach (or other leafy vegetable) to the saucepan and simmer for another 5 minutes, or until vegetables are tender. Meanwhile, in a heat-resistant serving bowl, dissolve the miso in 2 tablespoons of broth from the pot. Add the spring onion and sesame oil (if using). Remove the pot from the heat and carefully transfer the contents to the serving bowl. Garnish with shallots and serve immediately.

Note: For a tasty variation, substitute your favourite stock for the water. When adding the vegetables, use any other favourite, fast-cooking vegetables, such as zucchini, onions, bean sprouts, snow peas or chopped cabbage.

LENTIL AND VEGETABLE SOUP

(Makes 8 servings)

This hearty soup is easy to prepare and can be ready to eat in under an hour. The recipe can be halved if desired or the whole recipe can be made and part put in the freezer to be available for another meal.

8 cups water
2 cups dry lentils, washed and rinsed
1 can (400g) crushed tomatoes
1 large onion, chopped
Low-GI vegetables of choice (e.g. broccoli)
3–4 cloves garlic, minced
$^1/_4$ cup Bragg Liquid Aminos (see Resources) OR organic soy sauce OR
   bouillon
1 tablespoon dried basil
1 tablespoon ground cumin
1 tablespoon balsamic vinegar

Bring the water to a boil in a large saucepan over high heat. Add the lentils, tomatoes, onion, garlic, liquid aminos (or soy sauce or bouillon), basil, cumin and vinegar. Return to the boil, then reduce the heat to low. Simmer, uncovered, for 30 minutes. Add vegetables and continue simmering for 15 minutes, or until lentils and vegetables are tender.

BORSCHT

4 cups water
4 cups beetroot, peeled and cut into chunks or shredded
$1/2$ cup finely diced onion
2 teaspoons olive oil
1 tablespoon apple cider vinegar or lemon juice
1 clove garlic
2 bay leaves
Pepper
$1/3$ cup freshly chopped dill
$1/2$ cup finely chopped fresh parsley

Bring water to simmer. Add beetroot, onions, garlic and seasonings and simmer gently for about 15 minutes. Add oil, vinegar or lemon juice. Continue simmering for about 10 minutes. Remove from heat. Stir in parsley and dill. Serve hot. Add some natural yoghurt to garnish.

VEGETABLE BROTH

Make your own vegetable broth from (but not limited to) the following:

2 sliced potatoes
1 cup carrots
1 cup other vegetables such as cabbage or broccoli (choose organic where possible)
Water (filtered or spring) to cover the vegetables

Add potatoes, carrots and other vegetables of choice to a saucepan and cover with water. Gently simmer the vegetables on a low heat for about 30 minutes. Strain and drink the liquid.

Salads

ASPARAGUS AND LENTIL SALAD WITH TOMATO–LEMON DRESSING

(Makes 6 servings)

Asparagus and lentils, packed with folate, make a delicious salad when
  tossed in a tomato–lemon dressing
1 cup lentils
700g asparagus, trimmed and cut into 2.5 cm lengths (5 cups)
1 can (170ml) tomato juice
3 tablespoons fresh lemon juice
2 tablespoons organic extra-virgin olive oil
1 tablespoon organic Dijon mustard
3/4 teaspoon Celtic sea salt
1 punnet cherry tomatoes, halved
1 large red onion, diced
8 cups shredded spinach

Prep time: 25 minutes

Cook lentils for 30 minutes in a large pot of boiling salted water. Add
asparagus to pot and cook 2 to 3 minutes or until asparagus and
lentils are tender. Meanwhile, in a large bowl, whisk together tomato
juice, lemon juice, oil, mustard and salt. Add lentil mixture, toss well.
Cool to room temperature, add tomatoes, onion and spinach, and
toss again.

AVOCADO AND ROCKET SALAD WITH BASIL MUSTARD VINAIGRETTE

(Makes 4 servings)

Dressing:
1/4 cup flaxseed oil
1/4 cup balsamic vinegar
3 tablespoons chopped fresh basil leaves

2 teaspoons organic Dijon mustard
1 clove garlic, peeled and crushed
$1/4$ teaspoon salt
$1/8$ teaspoon pepper

Salad:
2 cups baby spinach
3 cups rocket
1 punnet cherry tomatoes
$1/2$ cup finely sliced Spanish (red) onion
1 avocado, cut into 1cm cubes

Prep time: 20 minutes

In a small jar, combine flaxseed oil, vinegar, basil, mustard, garlic, salt and pepper. Cover and shake until well combined. In a large salad bowl, combine spinach, rocket, tomatoes, onion, avocado and dressing. Toss to combine.

CHICKPEA AND BROCCOLI SALAD WITH FLAXSEED-TAHINI DRESSING

(Serves 4–6)

Dressing:
2 tablespoons flaxseed oil
3 tablespoons tahini
$1^1/2$ tablespoons lime juice
2 cloves garlic
2 tablespoons tamari
2 tablespoons water

Salad:
2 x 400g cans organic chickpeas, drained
2 cups broccoli florets, lightly steamed
$3/4$ cup chopped white or Spanish onion
1 cup thinly sliced radishes
Salt and pepper to taste

Combine all ingredients for the dressing in a blender or food processor and process to an even consistency. In a large bowl, toss chickpeas, broccoli, onion and radishes together with tahini dressing. Season with salt and pepper and chill thoroughly before serving.

BEETROOT AND ROCKET SALAD WITH LEMON–GINGER DRESSING

(Serves 4)

The nuttiness of rocket and the bite of the ginger dressing go really well together with the rich, earthy flavour of the beetroots.

8 medium beetroots (5 cm size)
100–150g baby rocket
1 cup sunflower sprouts
1 cup mung bean sprouts
1 tablespoon black sesame seeds (or regular sesame seeds)

Dressing:
1 tablespoon ginger, minced
1 spring onion top, thinly sliced
$1/2$ teaspoon lemon zest
2 tablespoons lemon juice
$1/4$ teaspoon garlic, minced
$1/4$ cup extra-virgin olive oil
2 tablespoons balsamic vinegar

Wash beetroots and steam or boil them until tender (up to 40 minutes), then cool and chill. Place all dressing ingredients in a blender and purée. Peel chilled beetroots and slice thinly. Divide rocket among four salad plates. Overlap beets in a ring around the rocket. Place sprouts in the centre of the ring and top with sesame seeds. Drizzle with dressing.

SPINACH AND EGG SALAD WITH SPROUTS, MUSHROOMS AND RADISHES

(Serves 4)

6 cups loosely packed organic spinach, washed and dried
1 cup mixed sprouts (clover, mung bean or snow pea)
1 cup sliced button mushrooms or other mushrooms
$1/2$ cup sliced radishes
2 organic hardboiled eggs, peeled and sliced finely

Gently toss all ingredients together and serve with a dressing of choice.

BEETROOT AND GREEN SALAD

250g fresh cooked beetroots
2 tablespoon chopped walnuts
Bed of rocket or cos lettuce

Toss and serve with favourite dressing.

ROCKET, WALNUT AND APPLE SALAD

Salad:
2 apples, peeled, cored and cut into chunks
1 bunch rocket
5 teaspoons chopped walnuts
50g goat's or sheep's milk feta, crumbled

Dressing:
2 tablespoons walnut oil
2 tablespoons olive oil
3 tablespoons balsamic vinegar
Salt and pepper to taste

Toss the salad ingredients and drizzle with the dressing.

PAWPAW AND CARROT SALAD

2 cups of lettuce, such as Cos
1 grated carrot
1/2 pawpaw, diced

Toss salad ingredients together. Mix 1 tablespoon raspberry vinegar and 1 tablespoon extra-virgin olive oil and fresh lemon juice and drizzle over the top.

TUNA, EGG AND BEAN SALAD

100g tuna (in spring water)
2 free-range hardboiled eggs
1 tomato
3 olives
2 cups of lettuce and other leafy greens
90g cooked mixed beans

Toss and drizzle with dressing of choice.

EDAMAME SALAD WITH HERBS

4 large garlic cloves, unpeeled
1 bag (450–500g) organic shelled edamame (soybeans)
1/4 teaspoon salt
1 cup plain yoghurt
1/4 cup chopped fresh flat-leaf parsley
2 tablespoons finely diced red capsicum
1 tablespoon thinly sliced fresh basil
2 teaspoons balsamic vinegar
Cos lettuce leaves for serving

Roast the garlic in an ungreased skillet over medium heat, turning frequently until softened (they'll have dark splotches in spots) — about 15 minutes. Cool and slip off the papery skins. Boil the edamame beans in salted water to cover until tender, about 5 minutes. Drain. Mix the beans and remaining ingredients. Add sea salt to taste (usually about 1/2 teaspoon). Serve the salad on lettuce leaves.

ROCKET SALAD WITH FENNEL AND PINE NUTS

(Serves 6)

2 cups baby rocket
2 small fennel bulbs, thinly sliced
1 red capsicum, halved, thinly sliced
3/4 cup toasted pine nuts
2 tablespoons lemon juice
1 teaspoon finely grated lemon zest
2 cloves garlic, minced
1/2 cup organic extra-virgin olive oil
1/2 teaspoon freshly ground black pepper
1/3 cup grated parmesan cheese

In a large salad bowl, combine rocket, fennel, capsicum and pine nuts. In a small bowl, whisk remaining ingredients until well blended. Pour over salad and toss well.

THAI TOFU SALAD

2 cups cooked cabbage
1 tablespoon peanut sauce
1 tablespoon sunflower seeds
85g firm tofu
1/4 cup fresh coriander (for garnish)

Dressing:
2 medium tomatoes, sliced and topped with 2 minced garlic cloves
2 tablespoons freshly chopped basil
1 tablespoon balsamic vinegar

Cut 85g of firm tofu into cubes and heat in a non-stick pan for 5 minutes. Place the cooked cabbage, peanut sauce and sunflower seeds in a saucepan. Heat over a medium heat for about two minutes (until warmed through, but still crunchy). Top with 1/4 cup chopped fresh coriander and serve.

ROASTED CAPSICUM, TOMATO AND CHICKPEA SALAD

(Serves 6)

Pumpkin seed oil has a rich, nutty flavour. If you can't find it, substitute dark sesame oil. Hulled pumpkin seeds are sold in most health-food stores, sometimes labelled 'pepitas'.

3 red capsicums, cut lengthwise into flat panels
1 clove garlic, peeled and halved
3 tablespoons balsamic vinegar
4 teaspoons pumpkin seed oil
$1/2$ teaspoon sea salt
1 punnet cherry tomatoes, halved
1 cup cooked chickpeas (rinsed and drained if canned)
4 tablespoons toasted hulled pumpkin seeds
4 cups Cos lettuce cut into bite-sized pieces

Prep time: 25 minutes

Preheat the grill. Place capsicum pieces, skin-side up, on rack and grill 10cm from heat for 10 minutes or until skin is charred. Remove capsicums, but leave grill on. When capsicums are cool enough to handle, peel and cut into 1cm strips. In a large bowl, whisk together vinegar, oil and salt. Add capsicum strips, tomatoes, chickpeas and pumpkin seeds and toss to combine. Add lettuce, toss again.

CHICKEN SALAD NIÇOISE STYLE

(Serves 4)

200g green beans, cut into 5cm pieces
450g skinless, boneless free-range chicken breasts
$3/4$ teaspoon salt
$1/2$ teaspoon oregano
$1/4$ teaspoon pepper
$1/3$ cup fresh lemon juice
1 tablespoon organic Dijon mustard
1 tablespoon extra-virgin olive oil
4 plum tomatoes cut into wedges
$1/4$ cup Kalamata or other olives, pitted
3 cups torn Cos lettuce leaves
2 tablespoons chopped fresh basil

Prep time: 30 minutes

In a large pot of boiling water, cook green beans for about 2 minutes or to between crisp and tender. Drain, rinse with cold water and drain again. Preheat the grill. Rub chicken with $1/2$ teaspoon of salt, $1/2$ teaspoon oregano and $1/4$ teaspoon pepper. Grill chicken for 4 minutes per side, or until cooked through. When cool enough to handle, cut chicken into thin diagonal slices. In a large bowl, whisk together remaining $1/4$ teaspoon salt, lemon juice, mustard and oil. Add green beans, chicken slices, tomatoes, olives, lettuce, and basil. Toss to combine.

GREEK SALAD

4 tomatoes, wedged or sliced
1 cucumber, seeded and sliced
1 red capsicum, seeded and sliced
1 small white onion, sliced finely
12 Kalamata olives
100g firm feta
$1/4$ cup olive oil
1 teaspoon dried oregano
$1/4$ cup parsley
Salt
Pepper
juice of 1 lemon

Chop tomatoes, cucumbers, capsicums, onion, olives and feta. In a small bowl whisk together oil, herbs, spices and the juice from the lemon. Drizzle dressing over salad.

LENTIL, GOAT'S CHEESE AND BEETROOT SALAD

(Serves 4)

3 cloves garlic, minced
1¹/₂ teaspoons grated lemon zest
1 teaspoon dried tarragon
³/₄ teaspoon salt
1¹/₂ cups lentils, washed and rinsed
¹/₃ cup fresh lemon juice
4 tablespoons extra-virgin olive oil
4 tablespoons organic Dijon mustard
1 capsicum, diced
1¹/₂ cups diced cooked beetroots
6 cups mixed greens (or substitute watercress or fresh spinach)
¹/₂ cup crumbled goat's cheese or feta
2 tablespoons coarsely chopped pecans

Prep time: 50 minutes

In a medium saucepan, combine 3 cups of water, the garlic, lemon zest, tarragon and salt, and bring to a boil over a high heat. Add lentils, reduce to a simmer, cover and cook 25 minutes, or until lentils are firm–tender. Drain any liquid remaining. In a medium bowl, combine lemon juice, oil and mustard. Add lentil mixture, capsicum and beetroot, tossing until well coated. Serve lentil mixture on a bed of greens and sprinkle with goat's cheese and pecans.

Salad dressings and sauces

THAI-STYLE FISH SAUCE

To give your fish added zing and interest you can make up this sauce and spread onto salmon or any other fish before cooking.

1 clove garlic, crushed
Small slice fresh ginger (finely grated)
2 chillies, deseeded and chopped
Juice and zest of 1 lime
Handful fresh coriander leaves
$^1/_4$ teaspoon sea salt
1 teaspoon sesame oil

Combine ingredients and whiz to a paste in a food processor. Spread onto the salmon or other fish fillets and bake in a hot oven or place under the grill until the fish is done.

SALSA

(Makes 6 servings)

This fresh salsa makes a great accompaniment to any piece of freshly cooked fish or chicken. You can even use it as a tasty topping for a plain omelette.

3–4 ripe tomatoes, diced or chopped finely
2 cloves garlic, minced
1 small red onion, finely chopped
1 jalapeño pepper, seeded and diced (wear plastic gloves when handling)
$^1/_2$ cup coriander leaves, chopped
Juice of 1 lime
Sea salt

In a medium bowl, combine the tomatoes, garlic, onion, pepper, coriander and lime juice. Season with salt to taste. Refrigerate until ready to serve.

AVOCADO SALSA

(Makes 2 servings)

$^1/_2$ avocado, diced small
1 large plump organic tomato
8–10 Kalamata olives, seeded and finely chopped
1 clove garlic, crushed
1 tablespoon finely chopped fresh basil
1 tablespoon finely chopped chives
1 tablespoon extra-virgin olive oil
1 teaspoon capers, drained
1 tablespoon lemon juice
Freshly ground salt and pepper to taste
1 jalapeño pepper, finely chopped (wear plastic gloves when handling)

In a small bowl combine all the ingredients and season with freshly ground salt and pepper to taste. Refrigerate until ready to serve.

TAHINI DRESSING

(Makes approximately 1 cup)

$^1/_2$ cup organic tahini
1–2 cloves garlic, crushed
$^1/_2$ cup lemon juice (plus extra)
1 teaspoon sea salt
filtered water

Whisk the first four ingredients together and refrigerate until ready to serve. It will thicken in the fridge, so you may need to add a little water or extra lemon juice to achieve a runny consistency.

TOMATO BASIL DRESSING

(Makes 4–6 servings)

Serve this light dressing over the freshest green salad.

$^1/_4$ **cup fresh basil leaves**
1 medium tomato
2–4 tablespoons balsamic or red wine vinegar
$^1/_2$ **cup extra-virgin olive oil**
$^1/_2$ **clove garlic, minced**
Salt to taste
Freshly cracked black pepper to taste

Combine all ingredients in a food processor. Blend until creamy. Adjust flavours if necessary.

FLAXSEED DRESSING

$^2/_3$ **cup flaxseed oil**
$^1/_4$ **cup balsamic vinegar or lemon juice**
1 teaspoon Dijon mustard
1 clove garlic, crushed
Fresh herbs
Ground pepper to taste

Place all ingredients in a jar and shake vigorously. Store in the fridge for up to two weeks.

GINGER MISO DRESSING

90 grams (^{1}/$_3$ cup) organic plain silken tofu
^{1}/$_3$ cup (80ml) organic soymilk
1 tablespoon fresh ginger, peeled and minced
1^1/$_2$ teaspoon tamari (wheat-free soy sauce)
1 teaspoon light miso
1 teaspoon Dijon mustard
1 tablespoon chopped coriander
1 tablespoon chopped spring onion

Combine the tofu, soymilk, ginger, tamari, mustard and miso in a blender. Process until just smooth and creamy. Transfer to a bowl and stir in the coriander and spring onion. Cover and refrigerate until ready to serve over salad. Use within two days.

Fish recipes

GRILLED RED SNAPPER WITH TOMATO SALSA

(Serves 4)

^{3}/$_4$ cup ripe Roma tomatoes
^{1}/$_4$ cup chopped onion
^{1}/$_4$ cup Kalamata olives, pitted and sliced
1 garlic clove, crushed
1^1/$_2$ tablespoons fresh chives, finely sliced
1^1/$_2$ tablespoons fresh basil, chopped
^{1}/$_2$ tablespoon fresh rosemary, chopped
2 tablespoons olive oil, divided
1 tablespoon drained capers
1^1/$_2$ teaspoons lemon juice
Salt and pepper to taste
4 red snapper fillets

In a medium bowl combine tomatoes, onion, olives, garlic, chives, basil, rosemary, 1 tablespoon olive oil, capers and lemon juice.

Cover and let rest at room temperature for about 30 minutes. Season with salt and pepper.

   Prepare a charcoal grill or heat a gas grill to high. Brush fillets with remaining olive oil. Season with salt and pepper. Grill fillets for 3–4 minutes. Place on individual plates and top with salsa.

ROASTED OCEAN TROUT WITH PESTO CRUST

6 ocean trout fillets, rinsed and patted dry
$1/2$ cup basil pesto
$1^1/2$ tablespoons coconut oil
1 shallot or 2 small spring onions, minced
500g baby spinach leaves, washed
Sea salt and freshly ground pepper to taste
6 cherry tomatoes

Preheat the oven to 200 degrees Celsius. Spread 2 tablespoons of pesto over the ocean trout fillets. In an ovenproof pan melt 2 teaspoons of coconut oil over high heat. Sear the ocean trout, pesto side down, for 2–3 minutes. Gently turn over the fillets with a long spatula. Place in the oven for 5–6 minutes until lightly cooked through. Add the remaining coconut oil and minced shallots to another skillet, stirring until the onion is translucent, or about 1 minute. Squeeze out any extra moisture from the spinach leaves and pat dry. Add the salt and pepper to the skillet and sauté quickly over high heat, or about 1–2 minutes. Divide the spinach onto serving plates as a bed for the ocean trout. Place the ocean trout fillet on top and garnish with the cherry tomatoes.

GRILLED SALMON WITH CHILLI CORIANDER PESTO

(Serves 4)

This recipe is great for casual entertaining as it can be assembled hours before-hand and grilled at the last minute.

4 salmon fillets or cutlets, skinned
Handful of fresh coriander, about 30g
1 red chilli, deseeded and roughly chopped
1 clove garlic, crushed
Grated zest and juice of 1 lime
$^1/_2$ teaspoon sea salt
2 tablespoons extra-virgin olive oil

 TIP

You can also spread the pesto on boneless chicken breasts, which will take 20–25 minutes to grill.

Remove any thick stalks from the coriander (small ones can be left on), roughly chop and place in the bowl of a food processor. Add the chilli, garlic, lime zest, juice and salt and whiz until the ingredients are well chopped. With the processor still running, pour in the olive oil until the mixture is a wet paste. (You can store the chilli coriander pesto in a jar in the fridge for several days.)

Preheat the grill to high. Place the salmon fillets on a baking sheet and spread one side with the pesto. You can cover and store them in the fridge at this stage if serving later. Depending on the strength of your grill and the thickness of the salmon, they should take 8–10 minutes to cook.

PUMPKIN SEED-CRUSTED SNAPPER

1/2 teaspoon coriander
1/4 cup raw pumpkin seeds, chopped
1/4 cup olive oil
2 fillets of snapper or other fish
1 lemon (juiced)
1 tablespoon parsley

Preheat the oven to 180 degrees Celsius. Add the coriander to the pumpkin seeds, then puree or roughly chop the seeds in a food processor, being careful to avoid a flour-like texture. Spread the olive oil over the bottom of the baking dish. Lightly coat the snapper with olive oil so that all sides of the fish are lightly coated. With one hand, spoon the chopped pumpkin seeds onto all sides of the fish while using the fingers of your other hand to pat the seeds onto the fish. Bake the fish for about 10–15 minutes or until done. When done, squeeze lemon juice onto each piece of fish and sprinkle with freshly chopped parsley.

BARRAMUNDI WITH LIME, GINGER AND SHIITAKE MUSHROOMS

(Serves 4 as a main course)

4 x 180g barramundi fillets
100g fresh shiitake mushrooms, sliced
3 teaspoons ginger, grated
3 tablespoons tamari (wheat-free soy sauce)
3 tablespoons lime juice
1 tablespoon toasted sesame seed oil
1 teaspoon sesame seeds, toasted
1/3 cup coriander, finely chopped

Prep time: 20 minutes

Partially fill a wok or saucepan with water and bring to the boil. Place a plate in a steamer (bamboo is ideal) or line the steamer with baking paper. Sit the steamer over the wok or saucepan so that the base does not touch the water. Arrange the mushrooms in the steamer and place the barramundi fillets on top of the mushrooms. Combine the ginger, tamari, lime juice, sesame seed oil and sesame seeds in a bowl. Spoon the sauce over the fish, sprinkle fish with coriander and cover with a lid. Steam for 10–12 minutes, or until the fish is opaque or flakes easily with a fork. Remove steamer and serve barramundi fillets and mushrooms, spooning any remaining sauce over the fillets.

BLUE-EYE COD, POACHED WITH SAFFRON, FENNEL AND TOMATO

(Serves 4)

1 tablespoon extra-virgin olive oil
1 onion, diced
1/2 bulb fresh fennel, diced
2 cloves garlic, finely sliced
1/2 teaspoon fennel seeds
1/2 cup white wine
3 cups fish stock
1/2 teaspoon saffron threads
2 large ripe tomatoes
4 x 180g blue-eye cod fillets
1 teaspoon sea salt
1 tablespoon fennel sprigs, from the fennel bulb

Prep time: 25 minutes

Preheat the oven to 180 degrees Celsius. Take a heavy roasting dish and preheat it to a moderate heat on top of the stove. Add 1 tablespoon olive oil, the onions, diced fennel, garlic and fennel seeds and cook gently, stirring occasionally until the onions are translucent and soft. Add the wine followed by the stock and the saffron threads. Cut the tomatoes in half across the centre and gently squeeze to remove the seeds, roughly chop and add to the roasting dish. Place the blue-eye cod fillets in the roasting dish, cover the pan tightly with foil and place in the oven. Use a spatula to turn the fish gently after 7 minutes and return to the oven for a further 3–4 minutes or until just cooked.

To serve, use a slotted spoon to place some of the vegetables in the centre of deep plates or wide bowls. Place the fish on top of the vegetables and spoon some of the cooking liquid over the fish. Scatter sprigs of fennel over each plate and serve immediately.

STEAMED SNAPPER WITH GINGER AND SHALLOTS
(Serves 4)

500g snapper fillets
8 spring onions
4cm fresh ginger, peeled
$^1/_2$ cup fresh coriander
2 tablespoons organic tamari (wheat-free soy sauce)
2 tablespoons extra-virgin olive oil
Juice of $^1/_2$ fresh lime
Juice of $^1/_2$ fresh lemon

Cut fish into 4cm pieces. Arrange fish on a small serving dish and put into steamer (bamboo works well). Shred the spring onions and ginger into thin matchsticks and scatter half of them over the fish, saving the rest for garnishing. Cover and cook gently over a moderate heat for five minutes or until fish flesh turns white. Place the fish on a serving plate, adding the remaining ginger, shallots and coriander, and sprinkle with tamari. Heat oil and lemon and lime juice until hot and pour over fish.

NUT-CRUSTED TUNA

(Serves 4)

This is a wonderful way of cooking fish steaks such as tuna or salmon. You can use almonds, walnuts or macadamia, hazel or pecan nuts.

4 x 150g boneless fish steaks
Extra-virgin olive oil (for greasing)
120g chopped nuts of choice (chop in a coffee grinder)
Sea salt to taste
Freshly ground black pepper to taste
2 teaspoons freshly chopped parsley
2 tablespoons melted coconut oil

Preheat the oven to 220 degrees Celsius. Grease a baking sheet with a little extra-virgin olive oil. Mix the chopped nuts together with the seasoning and put them on a plate. Melt the coconut oil in a pan and remove from heat. Dip the fish into the coconut oil, then into the nut mixture, pressing down to make sure the nuts hold. Place the nutted fish steaks onto the baking sheet and the put them into the oven for 8–10 minutes or until cooked through.

GRILLED MISO SALMON

(Serves 4)

$^{1}/_{2}$ cup (125ml) mirin (sweet rice cooking wine)
2 tablespoons minced fresh chives or spring onion tops
1 tablespoon yellow miso
1 tablespoon tamari (wheat-free soy sauce)
1 teaspoon tahini
1 teaspoon fresh ginger, peeled and minced
4 salmon fillets (150g each), skinned
2 tablespoons fresh coriander
1 teaspoon sesame seeds, toasted

In a shallow baking dish, whisk together the mirin, chives, miso, tamari, tahini and ginger. Add the salmon to the marinade and turn to coat. Cover and marinate in the refrigerator for 1–2 hours, turning the fish occasionally. Place a grill or a pan over high heat. Remove the fish from the marinade and pat dry. Discard the marinade. Return the grill or pan to the stove and when it is very hot place the fillets on it and cook, turning them carefully with a spatula, until grill-marked, firm to the touch and opaque in the centre, or for about four minutes on each side. Transfer the fillets to individual serving plates. Garnish with coriander and sesame seeds and serve immediately.

POACHED SEAFOOD IN LIME AND COCONUT DRESSING

400g mixed fresh seafood (prawns, scallops, fish)
500ml chicken stock (home-made)
1 spring onion, sliced
2 tablespoons coriander, chopped
1 teaspoon fresh mint, finely chopped
Juice of 2 limes
1/2 cup coconut milk
1 garlic clove, crushed
1 red chilli, diced
2 cups lettuce, shredded
1 teaspoon salt

Poach the seafood in a little chicken stock until just cooked (1–2 minutes). Spoon the seafood into a bowl of iced water until seafood is cool. Meanwhile, combine the rest of the ingredients (except the lettuce) to form a dressing. Drain the seafood from the water and add to the dressing. Cover and leave to marinate in the fridge for a minimum of 4 hours. To serve, place lettuce at the base of each serving bowl and pile over the seafood and dressing.

Chicken recipe

GRILLED CHICKEN BREASTS WITH MUSHROOMS

(Serves 4)

4 chicken breasts (organic/free range), skin off
$3/4$ cup Dijon marinade (see below)
1 cup wild rice (cooked)
$1^1/2$ tablespoons olive oil
1 cup wild mushrooms or shiitake mushrooms
1 yellow or brown onion, diced
1 garlic clove, minced
$1/8$ cup chopped fresh rosemary
$1/2$ cup toasted pine nuts (optional)

Dijon marinade:
$1/4$ cup Dijon mustard
$1/8$ cup lemon juice
$1/4$ cup red wine vinegar/balsamic vinegar
$1/2$ tablespoon dried tarragon
$1/8$ cup freshly chopped parsley
$1/8$ teaspoon Celtic sea salt
$1/3$ cup extra-virgin olive oil

To marinate the chicken: Combine all ingredients except olive oil into a medium-sized mixing bowl and mix well. Slowly drizzle in the olive oil while continuously whisking. Coat both sides of the chicken breasts with the marinade and put them into the fridge for about 4 hours. (Turn them over once while marinating.)

To cook the chicken: Gently stir fry or sauté the onions, garlic and mushrooms until the onions are translucent. Then grill the chicken until cooked through, or about five minutes on each side. Place the chicken on a plate, spoon over the mushrooms and onions. Sprinkle the freshly chopped rosemary and toasted pine nuts and serve with wild rice.

Red meat

MOROCCAN BEEF SALAD

650g eye fillet
$^1/_2$ teaspoon Celtic sea salt
$^1/_2$ teaspoon cracked black pepper
1 tablespoon olive oil (extra-virgin)
3 cups mixed salad leaves
$^1/_2$ cup chopped fresh coriander
6 small ripe tomatoes (quartered)
2 small red onions (cut into thin wedges)
zest of 1 orange

Dressing:
$^3/_4$ cup freshly squeezed orange juice
1 teaspoon paprika
1 teaspoon ground coriander
3 cloves garlic, crushed
1 small red chilli, chopped

Season beef with salt and pepper. Heat in a large frying pan with a little of the olive oil over high heat until brown all over. Transfer beef to an oven pan and roast at 220 degrees Celsius for 30 minutes (less if you want beef rare). Remove from oven and allow to cool. Combine salad ingredients in a bowl and place thinly sliced beef on top.

Dressing: Mix orange juice, spices, garlic, chilli and remaining olive oil and add salt and pepper to taste. Add dressing and orange zest to the salad and serve.

(Recipe courtesy of the Pro Health Clinic, Sydney)

Noodle dish

GARDEN-STYLE PRIMAVERA WITH RICE NOODLES

1 tablespoon extra-virgin olive oil
250g extra-firm tofu, cubed
1 cup cauliflower florets
1 cup broccoli florets
$^1/_2$ cup sliced red capsicum
1 teaspoon crushed garlic
$^2/_3$ cup of diced tomatoes, with juice
1 tablespoon fresh basil
$^1/_8$–$^1/_4$ teaspoon ground pepper
2 cups of rice noodles, cooked
3 tablespoons soy parmesan, grated (available at most good health-food stores)

Heat oil in large skillet. Add tofu, cauliflower, broccoli, red capsicum and garlic, and sauté for 3–5 minutes. Add tomato, basil and pepper, and simmer for 5–6 minutes. Add rice noodles and toss well. Top with soy parmesan and serve.

Vegetable dishes

SWEET POTATO MASH

(Serves 6)

2 medium sweet potatoes, approximately 1kg
1 pinch sea salt
$^1/_2$ cup soymilk or $^1/_2$ cup organic vanilla yoghurt
$^1/_2$ tablespoon chives, chopped

Peel sweet potatoes and place in pot. Cover with salted water and bring to the boil. Reduce heat and simmer for approximately 30 minutes or until soft. Drain potatoes well and place back into pot, add soymilk/yoghurt and chives and mash thoroughly.

ASPARAGUS WITH HAZELNUT GREMOLATA

(Serves 4)

Gremolata is a mixture of chopped parsley, garlic and lemon zest. It also complements steamed green beans, Brussels sprouts and broccoli.

500g asparagus, tough ends removed
1 clove garlic, minced
1 tablespoon chopped Italian (flat-leaf) parsley
1 tablespoon toasted hazelnuts, finely chopped
$1/4$ teaspoon finely grated lemon zest
2 teaspoons fresh lemon juice
1 teaspoon extra-virgin olive oil

TIP

A large saucepan fitted with a steamer is the best way to steam asparagus.

Put about 3cm of water in the bottom of the saucepan and bring it to a boil. Steam until the asparagus is tender–crisp, or for about 4 minutes. Remove from the steamer. In a large bowl combine the asparagus, chopped parsley, hazelnuts, garlic, lemon zest, lemon juice, olive oil and salt. Toss well to mix and coat the asparagus. It is a perfect accompaniment to any fish or chicken dish.

BROCCOLI STIR–FRY

Goes well with all fish dishes or grilled chicken.

1 tablespoon extra-virgin olive oil
1 onion
1 ginger chunk
4 cloves garlic
2 celery sticks
$1/2$ bunch broccoli or broccolini
3 shallots
$1/2$ cup chopped fresh basil
$1/2$ cup cashews (optional)
Celtic sea salt to taste

Gently fry onion, garlic, ginger and cashews in olive oil until onion becomes transparent. Add remaining vegetables and cook to your liking. Add basil, shallots and salt immediately before serving.

(Recipe courtesy of the Pro Health Clinic, Sydney)

QUINOA RISOTTO WITH ROCKET AND PARMESAN

(Serves 6)

Quinoa (pronounced *keen*-wah) is native to Peru and is much like wheat but higher in protein. It's available in most good health-food stores.

1 tablespoon extra-virgin olive oil
$1/2$ yellow onion, chopped
1 cup (185g) quinoa, well rinsed
$2^1/4$ cups vegetable or chicken stock or broth (no MSG)
2 cups rocket, chopped
1 small carrot, peeled and shredded finely
$1/2$ cup shiitake mushrooms, finely sliced
$1/4$ cup Parmesan cheese, grated
$1/2$ teaspoon Celtic sea salt
$1/4$ teaspoon freshly ground pepper

In a large saucepan, heat the olive oil over medium heat. Add the onion and sauté until soft and translucent, or about 4 minutes. Add the quinoa and garlic and cook for about a minute. Don't let the garlic brown. Add the stock and bring to the boil. Reduce the heat to low and simmer until the quinoa is almost tender to the bite but slightly hard in the centre, about 12 minutes. The mixture will be brothy. Stir in the rocket, carrot and mushrooms and simmer until the quinoa grains have turned from white to translucent, or about 2 minutes longer. Stir in the cheese and season with the salt and pepper. Serve immediately.

SWEET POTATO CAKES AND BAKED TOMATOES WITH ROCKET SALAD

430g orange sweet potatoes, peeled
1 egg, lightly beaten
1 tablespoon rice flour
$1/2$ tablespoon extra-virgin olive oil
4 tomatoes (halved)
$1/2$ teaspoon salt
$1/2$ teaspoon cracked black pepper
50g baby rocket
1 avocado, cut into wedges

Grate the sweet potato into a bowl and squeeze out excess moisture. Add the egg, flour, salt and olive oil to the sweet potato and gently mix. Shape the mixture into balls (approx 4 balls per heaped tablespoon of mixture) and flatten slightly before placing them on a non-stick baking tray that has been lightly (olive) oiled. Add tomato halves to the baking tray and sprinkle with salt and pepper. Bake in an oven heated to 200 degrees Celsius for 30 minutes. Serve cooked cakes and tomatoes with rocket and avocado wedges tossed together.

(Recipe courtesy of the Pro Health Clinic, Sydney)

Dips and snacks

ROASTED SOY NUTS

(Serves 6)

This easy-to-make crunchy treat tastes like dry roasted nuts but provides all the health benefits of soy.

1 cup dried soybeans
Salt or organic tamari / soy sauce

 TIP

For extra flavour, try sprinkling the soy nuts with onion powder or garlic powder or any favourite natural seasoning in addition to the salt or soy sauce.

Place the soybeans in a large bowl and cover with water. (They will more than double in volume, so make sure there is enough room in the bowl for the expansion and sufficient water to keep them covered.) Refrigerate the soaking soybeans overnight. Drain the soybeans in a colander and spread them between layers of paper towels to dry. Refrigerate for at least 1 hour. Preheat the oven to 130 degrees Celsius. Divide the soybeans onto two baking sheets. Roast for 1 hour or until lightly browned, turning occasionally with a spatula. Place the roasted soybeans in a large bowl and stir in the salt or tamari or soy sauce, to taste, while still hot.

CREAMY HUMMUS DIP

(Makes 8 servings)

Hummus makes a delicious and nutritious dip for fresh vegetables.

1 can (400g) organic chickpeas, rinsed and drained
2 spring onions, chopped into large pieces
4 cloves garlic
1 tablespoon tahini paste
3/4 teaspoon ground cumin
Juice of 1/2 lemon
2 teaspoons tamari or soy sauce
1/2 cup roasted red capsicum or 2 tablespoons fresh coriander (optional)
2 tablespoons extra-virgin olive oil

Place the chickpeas, spring onions, garlic, tahini, cumin, lemon juice, soy sauce, and roasted red capsicum or coriander (if using) in a blender or food processor. Purée until smooth.

VEGETABLE AND HERB TOFU DIP

Serve this dip with freshly sliced raw vegetables.

450–500g tofu
1 tablespoon brown onion, finely chopped
1 tablespoon fresh parsley, chopped
1 1/2 teaspoons dried basil
1 teaspoon salt
1 teaspoon organic tamari (wheat-free soy sauce)
1 teaspoon onion powder
1/2 teaspoon garlic powder
1/4 teaspoon ground cumin
1/4 teaspoon ground thyme
Pinch ground cayenne pepper
1 stick celery, finely chopped
1 carrot, finely chopped
1 green, red or yellow capsicum or any favourite raw vegetable, finely chopped (optional)

In a food processor or blender, blend the tofu until smooth (about 10 seconds). Add the onion, parsley, basil, salt, tamari, onion powder, garlic powder, cumin, thyme and ground red pepper. Process on pulse until just combined, or about 5 seconds. Place in a plastic container, and stir in the celery, carrot and capsicum or other vegetable (if using). Cover and refrigerate overnight to allow flavours to meld. Before serving, add more seasoning to taste because tofu continues to absorb flavour as it sits.

ALMOND, COCONUT AND BANANA POWER MUFFINS

1 cup almond meal
1/2 cup sunflower seeds
1/4 cup virgin coconut oil (available from most good health-food stores; if solid, melt slowly over low heat before use)
2 mashed bananas
2 organic eggs
1/2 cup whey protein
1/2 cup grated coconut
1 cup brown rice flour
1 teaspoon baking powder
1 cup soymilk/rice milk
1–2 tablespoons xylitol (optional)

Preheat oven to 200 degrees Celsius if a regular oven, or 170 degrees if fan forced. Combine all dry ingredients in a large bowl and whisk well. Combine all wet ingredients, including the mashed bananas, in a separate bowl. Add the wet ingredients to the dry ingredients and mix well. If the batter is too dry, add some more soy milk. Spoon into non-stick muffin baking tins or into paper muffin cups. Sprinkle tops with almond flakes or shredded coconut for decoration. Bake for approximately 30 minutes. Allow to cool, then keep in the fridge.

(Recipe courtesy of the Pro Health Clinic, Sydney)

Desserts

SPICY FRUIT COMPOTE

(Makes 6 servings)

Fruity and intensely seasoned, this compote provides the perfect antidote to a sweet craving.

1 orange, quartered
2 cups apple cider
1 teaspoon ground cinnamon
$1/2$ teaspoon ground nutmeg
$1/4$ teaspoon ground ginger
$1/8$ teaspoon ground cloves
4 dried, pitted prunes
1 apple, cored and cut into chunks
1 cup fresh or canned and drained pineapple chunks
2 fresh peaches, cut into slices, or 2 cups frozen and thawed peach slices
$1/2$ cup non-fat plain yoghurt (optional)

Chop one quarter of the orange, including the peel. Put the chopped orange, apple cider, cinnamon, nutmeg, ginger, cloves, and 4 prunes in a blender or food processor and process until smooth. Peel and coarsely chop the remaining 3 orange quarters. In a large saucepan over high heat, bring the blended mixture, chopped orange, apple, and remaining prunes to a boil. Reduce the heat to low, cover and simmer for 5 minutes, stirring occasionally. Add the pineapple and peaches to the pan and remove from the heat. Serve hot or refrigerate to serve cold. Top with a dollop of natural yoghurt (if using). Add some chopped nuts such as walnuts or pecans.

BAKED PEACHES WITH RICOTTA

(Serves 6)

6 large peaches
300g ricotta cheese
1 tablespoon clear organic honey
4 tablespoons crushed walnuts or macadamia nuts

Preheat the oven to 220 degrees Celsius. Cut the peaches in half and remove the stones. Line a baking dish with baking paper and place the peaches cut side up on the tray. Roast the peaches in a pre-heated oven for about 15–20 minutes or until the peaches are just tender. Let peaches cool slightly. Place them on plates and top with ricotta cheese, sprinkle with ground nuts and drizzle with honey.

GRILLED FRESH FIGS WITH MACADAMIA NUTS AND RICOTTA

Cut a cross across the top of whole figs and fill them with finely chopped macadamia nuts. Grill under a hot grill for five minutes and serve with fresh ricotta. Sweeten with a little raw honey if desired.

PEACHES WITH TOASTED MACADAMIA NUTS AND ALMOND CREAM

50g or about a $1/4$ cup macadamia nuts
4 peaches
1 tablespoon brown rice syrup
almond cream (see following recipe)

Spread nuts on oven tray and roast at 180 degrees Celsius for about 5 minutes or until golden. Cool for 10 minutes, then chop coarsely. Slice peaches and arrange on plates. Drizzle brown rice syrup over the top, sprinkle with macadamia nuts and drizzle over almond cream.

ALMOND CREAM

(Makes about 2 cups and keeps for several days when refrigerated)

$^3/_4$ cup water (185ml) filtered or spring water
95g plain organic yogurt or soy yogurt
1$^1/_2$ cups (150g) almond meal
1 tablespoon raw honey

Place the almond meal, water, honey and yogurt in a jug and use a hand blender to mix until the consistency of thickened pouring cream. Or place in a blender and blend until combined well.

MIXED FRESH BERRIES WITH GINGER SAUCE

(Serves 6)

Sauce:
500g (or 4 cups) strawberries, hulled and halved
$^1/_4$ cup freshly squeezed orange juice
$^1/_2$ teaspoon vanilla essence
3 tablespoons chopped crystallised ginger

Berries:
2 cups blackberries or other berries in season
1 cup raspberries
1 cup red currants
Fresh mint leaves for garnishing

To make the sauce, combine the strawberries, orange juice, vanilla essence and ginger in a blender. Process until just blended. Pass the purée through a fine-mesh sieve placed over a small bowl, pressing on the solids with a spatula or the back of a wooden spoon to extract all the juice. In a large bowl, toss together all the berries, including the red currants, mixing well. Transfer to a serving bowl or individual bowls. Spoon the ginger sauce over the berries and garnish with mint.

Notes

1   Wahlqvist, Mark, et al., 'Skin Wrinkling: Can Food Make a Difference'?
    Journal of the American College of Nutrition, vol. 20, no. 1, February 2001,
    pp. 71–80.

2   Allure readers poll, 'Body News', *Allure* magazine, June 2002.

3   Furnham, A., et al., University College London, 'Facial Attraction', *Allure* magazine, June 2002, p. 132.

4   Gotting, Peter, 'Rise of the Metrosexual', the *Age*, 11 March 2003.

5   Wahlqvist, Mark, et al., 'Skin Wrinkling: Can Food Make a Difference?'
    Journal of the American College of Nutrition, vol. 20, no. 1, February 2001,
    pp. 71–80.

6   Hilton, Lisette, 'Anti-ageing: The Other Half of a Surgeon's Offering:
    Comprehensive Approach Includes Nutrition', Diet, Exercise, *Cosmetic
    Surgery Times*, September 2004, pp. 22–4.

7   Dr Richard Glogau, interview with the author, 12 February 2005.

8   Foreman, Judy, 'Moisturiser Madness', *My Health Sense*, October 2001.
    Published at: www.myhealthsense.com Judy Foreman is a nationally syndicated US health columnist.

9   As above.

10 Blumberg, Dr Jeffrey, quoted by Paula Begoun, 'Antioxidants and Free
    Radical Damage', published at
    www.cosmeticscop.com/learn/article.asp?PAGETYPE=SKIN

11 Kligman, Albert M., MD, PhD, 'Dialogue with a mentor', *Dermatology Times*,
    1 September 2004, published at www.dermatologytimes.com

12 Baird-Murray, Kathleen, How to be Beautiful: *The Thinking Woman's Guide
    to Looking Good*, Vermillion, London, 2002.

13 Abell, Alicia, 'Hope in a Jar: Cosmetics Make Lots of Anti-aging Promises, But
    What Really Works?' *Washingtonian Online*, February 2004.

14 Smith, Timothy J., MD, *Renewal: The Anti-aging Revolution*, Rodale Press,
    Pennsylvania, 1998, p. 287.

15 Podda, M., Grundmann-Kollmann, M., et al., 'Low molecular weight antioxidants and their role in skin ageing', *Clinical & Experimental Dermatology*,
    vol. 26, no. 7, October 2001, pp. 578–82.

16 Prior, L. Ronald, et al., 'Lipophilic and Hydrophilic Antioxidant Capacities of
    Common Foods in the United States', *Journal of Agriculture and Food
    Chemistry*, vol. 52, no. 12, June 2004, pp. 4026–37.

17 Bland, Jeffrey, PhD, *The 20-Day Rejuvenation Diet Program*, Keats publishing, Connecticut, 1998, p. 96.

18   Legards, Jean-Francois, et al., 'Assessment of Lifestyle Effects on the Overall Antioxidant Capacity of Healthy Subjects,' *Environmental Health Perspective*, vol. 110, no. 5, May 2002, pp. 479–86.

19   Virginia, Worthington, 'Nutritional Quality of Organic Versus Conventional Fruits, Vegetables, and Grains,' *Journal of Alternative and Complementary Medicine*, vol. 7, no. 2, April 2001, pp 161–73.

20   Mitchell, A. E., et al., 'Comparison of the total phenolic and ascorbic acid content of freeze-dried and air dried marionberry, strawberry, and corn grown using conventional, organic, and sustainable agricultural practices', *Journal of Agricultural and Food Chemistry*, vol. 51, no. 5, February 2003, pp. 1237–41.

21   Pryme, I., and R. Lembcke, 'In vivo studies on possible health consequences of genetically modified food and feed — with particular regard to ingredients consisting of genetically modified plant materials'. *Nutrition and Health magazine*, vol. 17, 2003, pp. 1–8.

22   Wolff, M. S., et al., 'Blood level of organochlorine residues and risk of breast cancer', *Journal of the National Cancer Institute*, vol. 85, 1993, pp. 648–52.

22a Colborn, T., *Our Stolen Future*, Dutton Books (Penguin Group), New York, 1996, pp 54-85.

23   Schwartz, Steven J., et al., 'Carotenoid bioavailability is higher from salads ingested with full fat than with fat-reduced salad dressings as measured with electrochemical detection', *American Journal Clinical Nutrition*, vol. 80, August 2004, pp. 396–403.

24   Wahlqvist, Mark, et al., 'Skin Wrinkling: Can Food Make a Difference'? *Journal of the American College of Nutrition*, vol. 20, no. 1, February 2001, pp. 71–80.

25   Lyketsos, Constantine G., 'Should pregnant women avoid eating fish? Lessons from the Seychelles,' *The Lancet*, vol. 361. no. 9370, May 2003, p. 1667.

26   Kushi, Avelin, *Diet For Natural Beauty: Natural Anti-aging Formula for Skin and Hair Care*, Japan Publications, New York, 1991, p. 50

27   Challem, Jack, *The Inflammation Syndrome*, John Wiley and Sons, New Jersey, 2003, p. 44.

28   Cordain, L, et al, 'Modulation of immune function by dietary lectins in rheumatoid arthritis', *British Journal of Nutrition*, vol. 83, 2000, pp. 207–17.

28a Cordain, L., PhD, *The Paleo Diet: Lose Weight and Get Healthy by Eating the Food You Were Designed to Eat*, John Wiley & Sons, New York, 2002, p. 91.

29   Thomas, Regan, et al., 'Modulation of Cutaneous Aging With Calorie Restriction in Fischer 344 Rats', *Archives of Facial Plastic Surgery*, vol. 7, Jan–Feb 2005, pp. 12–16.

30   McBride, Judy, 'High ORAC foods may slow ageing', *Agricultural Research* magazine, vol. 47, no. 2, February 1999.

31 Vallejo, F. A. Tomás-Barberán and C. García-Viguera, 'Phenolic compound contents in edible parts of broccoli inflorescences after domestic cooking', *Journal of the Science of Food and Agriculture*, vol. 83, no. 14, October 2003, pp. 1511–16.

32 Lubec, G., et al., 'Amino acid Isomerisation and Microwave Exposure', *The Lancet*, vol. 2, no. 8676, 1989, pp. 1392–93.

33 Valentine, Tom, 'The Hidden Hazards of Microwave Cooking', *Nexus* magazine, vol. 2, no. 24, April/May 1995. Originally published in *Acres* magazine (US), April 1994.

34 Watson, R., et al., 'Carotenoid Supplementation Reduces Erythema in Human Skin After Simulated Solar Radiation Exposure', *Experimental Biology and Medicine*, vol. 223, no. 2, February 2000, pp. 170–74.

35 Amblard, P., et al., 'Low doses of zinc gluconate for inflammatory acne', *Acta Dermatovener* (Stockholm), vol. 69, 1989, pp. 541–3.

36 Wahlqvist, Mark, et al., 'Skin Wrinkling: Can Food Make a Difference?' *Journal of the American College of Nutrition*, vol. 20, no. 1, February 2001, pp. 71–80.

37 Synnott, Amy, 'Buying Face Time Wrinkle creams, Botox, lasers — our guide to the mountain of youth-promising skin treatments out there,' *Instyle* magazine, February 2002, p. 149.

38 Biesalski, H. K., and U. C. Obermueller-Jevic, 'UV light, beta-carotene and human skin — beneficial and potentially harmful effects', *Archives of Biochemistry and Biophysics*, vol. 389, no. 1, 2001, pp. 1–6.

39 Heinrich U., et al., 'Supplementation with beta-carotene or a similar amount of mixed carotenoids protects humans from UV-induced erythema', *Journal of Nutrition*, vol. 133, no. 1, January 2003, pp. 98–101.

40 Packer, Lester, and Carol Coleman, *The Antioxidant Miracle*, John Wiley & Sons, New York, 1999.

41 Garg A., et al, 'Psychological Stress Perturbs Epidermal Permeability Barrier Homeostasis', *Archives of Dermatology*, vol. 137, 2001, pp. 53-59.

42 Chopra, Deepak, MD, and David Simon, *Grow Younger, Live Longer: Ten Steps to Reverse Ageing*, Three Rivers Press, New York, 2001, p. 47.

43 Maclean, C. R., et al., 'Altered responses of cortisol, GH, TSH, and testosterone to acute stress after four months' practice of Transcendental Meditation (TM)', presented at the New York Academy of Sciences meeting on Brain Corticosteroid Receptors: Studies on the Mechanism, Function, and Neurotoxicity of Corticosteroid Action, Arlington, VA, 2–5 March 1994; Hoffman, J. W., et al., 'Reduced sympathetic nervous system responsivity associated with the relaxation response,' *Science*, vol. 38, 1989, pp. 15–21; Infante, J. R., et al., 'Catecholamine levels in practitioners of the transcendental meditation technique', *Physiology and Behavior*, vol. 71, no. 1–2, 2001, pp. 141–6.

44   Stein, Joel, 'Just Say Om,' *Time Magazine*, 4 August 2004.

45   MacLean, C., et al., 'Effects of the Transcendental Meditation program on adaptive mechanisms: changes in hormone levels and responses to stress after 4 months of practice', *Psychoneuroendocrinology*, vol. 22, no. 4, 1997. pp. 277–95; Glaser, J. L., et al., Elevated serum dehydroepiandrosterone (DHEA) sulphate levels in practitioners of transcendental meditation TM and TM-Sidhi programs', *Journal of Behavioral Medicine*, vol. 15, 1992, pp. 327–41.

46   Elsen, B. D., et al., 'Physiological changes in yoga meditation', *Psychophysiology*, vol. 14, 1977, pp. 52–7; Wallace, R. K., 'Physiological effects of transcendental mediation', *Science*, vol. 167, no. 926, 1970, pp. 1751–4.

47   Wallace, R. K., 'The effects of transcendental mediation and TM-Sidhi program on the aging process', *International Journal of Neuroscience*, vol. 16, pp. 53–8.

48   Khalsa, S. B., Treatment of chronic insomnia with yoga: a preliminary study with sleep-wake diaries', Applied Psychophysiology Biofeedback, vol. 29, no. 4. December 2004, pp. 269–78.

49   'Sex "key" to stay young', BBC online, 10 October 2000, published at: www.news.bbc.co.uk/1/hi/scotland/965045.stm

50   Van Cauter, E., et al., 'Alterations of circadian rhythmicity and sleep in aging. endocrine consequences', *Hormone Research*, vol. 49, no. 3–4, 1998, pp. 147–52.

51   Chrousos, G. P., et al., 'Chronic insomnia is associated with nyctohemeral activation of the hypothalamic-pituitary-adrenal axis: clinical implications', *Journal of Clinical Endocrinology & Metabolism*, vol., 86, no. 8, pp. 3787–94.

52   Coren, S., Sleep *Thieves: An Eye-opening Exploration into the Science and Mysteries of Sleep*, Free Press, New York, 1996.

53   Dement, William, PhD, *The Promise of Sleep*, Delacorte Press, New York, 1999.

54   Higuchi S., et al., 'Effects of VDT tasks with a bright display at night on melatonin, core temperature, heart rate, and sleepiness', *Journal of Applied Physiology*, vol. 94, no. 5, 2003, pp. 1773–6.

55   Somer, Elizabeth, *The Origin Diet: How Eating Like Our Stone Age Ancestors Will Maximize Your Health*, Owl Books, New York, 2001, p. 17.

56   Erasmus, Udo, *Fats That Heal, Fats That Kill: The Complete Guide to Fats, Oils, Cholesterol and Human Health*, Alive Books, Burnaby, B.C., Canada, 1993, p. 37.

57   Kushi, Avelin, Diet For Natural Beauty: *Natural Anti-aging Formula for Skin and Hair Care*, Japan Publications, New York, 1991, p. 60.

58   Munch, G., et al., 'Influence of advanced glycation end-products and AGE-inhibitors on nucleation-dependent polymerization of beta-amyloid peptide', *Biochimica et Biophysica Acta (International Journal of Biochemistry,*

Biophysics and Molecular Biology), vol. 1360, no. 1, 1997, pp. 17–29; Thome, J., et al., 'New hypothesis on etiopathogenesis of Alzheimer syndrome. Advanced glycation end products (AGEs)', *Nervenarzt*, vol. 67, no. 11, 1996, pp. 924–9.

59 Sajithlal, G. B., et al., 'Advanced Glycation End products induce cross-linking of collagen in vitro', *Biochimica Biophysica Acta*, vol. 1407, 1998, pp. 215–24.

60 Cordain, L., et al., 'Acne Vulgaris. A Disease of Western Civilization', *Archives of Dermatology*, vol. 138, no. 12, December 2002, pp. 1584–90.

61 Jee, Sun Ha, et al., 'Fasting Serum Glucose Level and Cancer Risk in Korean Men and Women,' *Journal of the American Medical Association*', vol. 293, January 2005, pp. 194–202.

62 Maher, T. J, and R. J. Wurtman, 'Possible Neurologic Effects of Aspartame, a Widely Used Food Additive', *Environmental Health Perspectives*, vol. 75, 1987, pp. 53–7.

63 Blaylock, Russell L., *Excitotoxins: The Taste That Kills*, Health Press, Santa Fe, New Mexico, 1994.

64 Kenton, Leslie, *New Joy of Beauty: The Complete Guide to Lasting Energy and Good Looks*, Vermillion, London, 1995, p. 77.

65 Butterer, Karmen, 'The Clear Skin Diet,' *Self* magazine, March 2001, p. 170–74.

66 Editors of Prevention Health Books, *Prevention's Best Anti-Aging Secrets*, St Martins, New York, 2001, p. 9.

67 Cordain, L., et al., 'Dissociation of the glycaemic and insulinaemic responses to whole and skimmed milk', *British Journal of Nutrition*, vol. 93, 2005, pp. 175–7. Ostman, E. M., et al., 'Inconsistency between glycemic and insulinemic responses to regular and fermented milk products', *American Journal of Clinical Nutrition*, vol. 74, 2001, pp. 96–100.

68 Paula Begoun, Wrinkles/Aging Skin; 'Antioxidants and Free Radical Damage', March/April 2002, published at: http://www.cosmeticscop.com/learn/dearpaula.asp?type=category&selCategory=4&btnGo=GO&type=category&txtKeywords=

69 Boyd, A. S., et al., 'Cigarette smoking: Associated elastotic changes in the skin', *Journal of the American Academy of Dermatology*, vol. 41 1999, pp. 23–6.

70 James, Kat, *The Truth About Beauty*, Beyond Words, Oregon, 2003, p. 158.

71 Centres for Disease Control and Prevention, 'Eighty-eight percent of non-smokers show signs in their blood of cotinine', *Allure* magazine, July 2002, p. 88.

72 Holick, Michael, *The UV Advantage: How to Harness the Power of the Sun for Your Health*, I Books, New York, 2004.

73 Partie Lange, Diane, *Allure* magazine, 'Tanning Beds' Effects', October 2001, p. 154.

74   Larsen, Hans R., MSc, 'Sunscreens: Do They Cause Skin Cancer'?
     International Journal of Alternative & Complementary Medicine, vol. 12, no.
     12, December 1994, pp. 17–19.

75   Garland, Cedric F., et al, 'Could sunscreens increase melanoma risk'?
     American Journal of Public Health, vol. 82, no. 4, April 1992, pp. 614–15;
     Garland, Cedric. F., et al., 'Rising trends in melanoma. A hypothesis concern-
     ing sunscreen effectiveness', *Annals of Epidemiology*, vol. 3, no. 1, 1993, p.
     103–10; Garland, Cedric F., et al, 'Effects of sunscreens on UV radiation-
     induced enhancement of melanoma growth in mice', *Journal of the National
     Cancer Institute*, vol. 86, no. 10, 1994, pp. 798–801.

76   BBC Health, 'Sunscreens may be toxic', Norwegian Radiation Protection
     Authority study, October 2000, published at:
     www.news.bbc.co.uk/1/hi/health/956342.stm

77   Schlumpf, Margret, et al., 'In Vitro and in Vivo Estrogenicity of UV Screens',
     Environmental Health Perspectives, vol. 109, no. 3, March 2001, pp. 239–44.

78   Liu, Guangming, et al., 'Omega 3 but not omega 6 fatty acids inhibit AP-1
     activity and cell transformation in JB6 cells', *Proceedings of the National
     Academy of Sciences of the United States of America (PNAS)*, vol. 98, no. 13,
     June 2001, pp. 7510–15.

79   Bain, C., et al., 'Diet and Melanoma: An exploratory case-control study',
     Annals of Epidemiology, vol. 3, no. 3, May 1993, pp. 235–8, Department of
     Social and Preventive Medicine, University of Queensland Medical School,
     Australia.

80   Williams, H., 'Melanoma with no sun exposure', *Lancet*, vol. 346, no. 8984,
     November 1995, p. 581.

81   Epel, Elissa S., et al., 'Accelerated telomere shortening in response to life
     stress', *Proceedings of the National Academy of Sciences of the United States of
     America (PNAS)*, vol. 101, no. 49, December 2004, pp. 17312–15.

82   Hung, L. M., et al., 'Cardioprotective effect of resveratrol, a natural antioxi-
     dant derived from grapes', *Cardiovascular Research*, vol. 47, 2000, pp.
     549–55.

83   Beiswanger, B. B., et al., 'The effect of chewing sugar-free gum after meals
     on clinical caries incidence', *Journal American Dental Association*, vol. 129,
     1998, pp. 1623–6.

84   McKinney, M., 'Dip into honey pot for good health', *Reuters Health*, 29 March
     2004.

Resources

ORGANIC DARK CHOCOLATE
Green and Black's
Available at most good health-food
shops and online at
www.greenandblacks.com

Kaoka
Available at most good health-food
shops and online at
www.lettucedeliver.com.au (but note
that it does contain milk protein).

Teeccino herbal coffees
Order online at www.teeccino.com

WHEY PROTEIN POWDER
**BioPure microfiltered whey protein con-
centrate from Metagenics**
Available at a selection of good health-
food shops. Or call Metagenics (freecall
1800 777 648) or go online at
www.metagenics.com.au to find a
health practitioner/retailer near you.

Whey protein isolate
Freecall 1800 247 757
www.aussiebodies.com.au
Also available at most good health-food
shops.

**PROTEIN CONCENTRATE (FOR DETOXI-
FICATION)**
Ultraclear protein powder
Ultraclear is a powdered beverage mix
which includes a specific blend of vitamins, minerals and other nutrients that
help support the body's detoxification
process. It is formulated with a rice
protein concentrate and has low allergy
potential. Available at a selection of
good health-food shops. Or call
Metagenics (freecall 1800 777 648) or
go online at www.metagenics.com.au

to find a health practitioner/retailer
near you.

Liquid aminos
Bragg Liquid Aminos is a certified non-
GMO liquid protein concentrate
derived from soybeans. It contains various essential and non-essential amino
acids in naturally occurring amounts.
Available at most good health-food
shops. For further information visit
www.bragg.com/products/
liquidaminos.html

NATURAL SWEETENER
Xylitol
Available at selected health-food stores
throughout Australia. Or purchase
online at www.sweetlife.com.au or
e-mail for further details.

MULTI-NUTRIENT REGIME
Multigenics Phyto Plus
www.metagenics.com.au

Life Extension Mix
www.lef.org

VITAMIN C
**Bio C from Blackmores — tablet or pow-
der form**
Tel: (02) 9951 0111
www.blackmores.com.au
Available from most health-food stores.

**C-Ultrascorb from Metagenics — tablet
or powder form**
Available at a selection of good health-
food shops. Or call Metagenics (freecall
1800 777 648) or go online at
www.metagenics.com.au to find a
health practitioner/retailer near you.

ALPHA-LIPOIC ACID
Metagenics Lipoic acid
Available at a selection of good health-
food shops. Or call Metagenics (freecall

1800 777 648) or go online at www.metagenics.com.au to find a health practitioner/retailer near you.

Bioceuticals Lipoic acid

Freecall: 1300 650 455 / (02) 9557 1688
www.bioceuticals.com.au
Available at selected health-food stores or contact Bioceuticals for your closest health provider or retailer.

Dr Vera's Formulations Lipoic acid

Tel: (07) 3868 0699
www.bioconcepts.com.au
Available from your health provider. Contact Bioconcepts for one nearest you.

Omega 3 fatty acids — EPA/DHA

Make sure the EPA/DHA you purchase is filtered or has undergone 'molecular distillation' to remove all heavy meals such as mercury and other pollutants.

Meta EPA/DHA from Metagenics

Available at a selection of good health-food shops. Or call Metagenics (freecall 1800 777 648) or go online at www.metagenics.com.au to find a health practitioner/retailer near you.

EPA/DHA Plus from Bioceuticals

Freecall: 1300 650 455 / (02) 9557 1688
www.bioceuticals.com.au
Available at selected health-food stores or contact Bioceuticals for the closest health practitioner/retailer.

COQ10

CoQ10–33 from Metagenics

Available at a selection of good health-food shops. Or call Metagenics (freecall 1800 777 648) or go online at www.metagenics.com.au to find a health practitioner/retailer near you.

CoQ10 100st 60 softgels from Bioceuticals

Freecall: 1300 650 455 / (02) 9557 1688

www.bioceuticals.com.au
Available at selected health-food stores or contact Bioceuticals for your closest health provider or retailer.

ACETYL L-CARNITINE

N-Acetyl Carnitine from Metagenics

Available at a selection of good health-food shops. Or call Metagenics (freecall 1800 777 648) or go online at www.metagenics.com.au to find a health practitioner/retailer near you.

Acetyl L-carnitine from Dr Vera's Formulations

Tel: (07) 3868 0699
www.bioconcepts.com.au

Acetyl L-carnitine powder from Musashi

www.thexton.com.au

SPIRULINA

Lifestream organic spirulina — tablets or powder

Hawaiian Pacifica spirulina — tablets or powder

Available from most good health-food shops.

GRAPESEED EXTRACT

Grapeseed 6000 plus

Tel: (02) 9899 9099
www.eaglepharmaceuticals.com.au

Grapeseed extract

www.lef.org

MSM (METHYLSULFONYLMETHANE)

MSM powder

Eagle Pharmaceuticals
Tel: (02) 9899 9099
www.eaglepharmaceuticals.com.au
Pharma Foods
Freecall: 1300 362 440
www.pharmafoods.com.au

SELENIUM

Selenosol from Nutrition Care — liquid selenium

Traditional Medicine Supplies
Freecall: 1800 650 877
www.tradmed.com.au
Note: One drop = 10 micrograms of Selenium.
Practitioner-only range. However, many of these products are available through a naturopath or other health providers on staff at most good health-food stores. Alternatively call TMS for your closest health care provider or retailer.

CARNOSINE

Super Carnosine

www.lef.org

Probiotics

Look for Natren and Metagenics brands.

GREEN DRINKS

'Perfect food' by Garden of life

www.gardenoflife.com
May also be ordered online at www.lef.org or www.netriceuticals.com

ProGreens powder (265 grams) by Allergy Research Group

May be ordered through www.netriceuticals.com

WHOLEFOOD SUPPLEMENTS

Juice Plus+

www.juiceplus.com.au
Juice Plus+ is an excellent wholefood supplement that's backed by a large body of independent scientific research. A number of studies have shown that it increases the level of antioxidants in the blood and decreases the level of rancid fat molecules (lipid peroxides) among other things. Go to the website for more information.

GNLD (GOLDEN NEO-LIFE DIAMITE) INTERNATIONAL

PhytoDefense by GNLD.

PhytoDefense is a comprehensive wholefood supplement pack containing the supplements 'carotenoid complex', 'flavonoid complex' and 'cruciferous plus'. The carotenoids contain fruits and vegetables like carrots and tomatoes; flavonoids from foods such as grapes and citrus fruits; and cruciferous compounds from vegetables like broccoli and radishes.
www.gnld.com.au

OILS

Organic cold-pressed flaxseed oil from Stoney Creek

Tel: 03 5463 2340
www.stoneycreekoil.com.au
Available at most good health-food stores.

Organic cold-pressed flaxseed oil from Melrose

Available at most good health-food stores.

Virgin cold-pressed coconut oil

Make sure the coconut oil you buy is virgin and cold-pressed. Available at most good heath-food stores or purchase online at www.tropicaltraditions.com

ORGANICS

For information on organics in Australia visit www.australianorganic.com.au
Biological Farmers of Australia (BFA) provides an online directory of certified organic retailers, butchers and organic delivery services at www.bfa.com.au
For a directory of organic food deliveries and organic food shops go to www.ecoshop.com.au

Macro Wholefoods

Macro Wholefoods are Sydney's largest organic stores, with shops at Bondi Junction and Crows Nest. Both stores

offer a large range of products, including 100% certified organic fruits and vegetables, organic and biodynamic dairy goods, sugar-free natural snacks, herbs, supplements, sourdough and organic breads, gluten-free breads and pastas, organic breakfast cereals, soymilks and grain milks, environmentally friendly cleaning and pet products, bulk natural foods, books and magazines.
Bondi Junction tel: (02) 9389 7611
Crows Nest tel: (02) 9966 8788
www.macrowholefoods.com.au

Vibrant markets (Northern Beaches, Sydney)
Certified Organic Market
8 a.m. to 12 p.m. every Saturday
Manly West Public School
Hill Street
Balgowlah NSW 2093
Contact Danielle Neill for further information.
Tel: 0412 879 923
www.vibrantmarkets.com.au

ORGANIC DELIVERY SERVICES

NEW SOUTH WALES/ACT
Lettuce Deliver
One of Australia's longest running home delivery services, specialising in the delivery of certified organic fruit, vegetables, groceries and meat produce across Sydney.
Tel: (02) 9763 7337
Online shopping at
www.lettucedeliver.com.au

Dynamic Organics
Delivering certified organic fruit, vegetables and other groceries to most north shore and northern beach suburbs in Sydney.
Tel: (02) 9905 5553
Online shopping at
www.dynamicorganics.com

Sam the Butcher
Offers a wide selection of organic meats and poultry, along with other products which can be ordered online and delivered fresh, fast and straight to your door. Their organic meats and poultry are totally free of GMO (Genetically Modified Organisms), preservatives, hormones, growth promotants and other chemical nasties.
Sans Souci Store tel: (02) 9583 1144
Bondi Store tel: (02) 9389 1420
Beecroft Store tel: (02) 9484 7138
Naremburn tel: (02) 9437 1090
http://www.samthebutcher.com.au

Organics Harvest
Organics Harvest in Canberra stock an extensive product range of organics including fruit, vegetables and culinary herbs, grocery products and dry goods, dairy and non-dairy products, eggs, breads, flour, grains, beans, nuts, seeds, oils, tofu, snack foods, chocolates, cosmetics and baby foods.
Tel: (02) 6253 0444
www.organicsharvest.com.au

WESTERN AUSTRALIA
The Earth Market
The Earth Market in Perth is a wholefood store/café specialising in organic produce.
Tel: (08) 9382 2266

VICTORIA
The Green Line
The Green Line offers the largest range of certified organic and bio-dynamic products in Victoria. Home delivery to all Melbourne suburbs and country Victoria destinations. Orders may be placed online or by phone/fax.
Tel: (03) 9460 3999
www.greenlinedelivery.com.au

Organic Wholefooods

Melbourne's largest natural food retailer, with an extensive range of high-quality certified organic and biodynamic foods.
Tel: (03) 9384 0288
www.wholefoods.com.au

Passion Foods Eco-living

Stocking quality, naturally raised, organic and biodynamic fresh produce, chemical-free gourmet foods and earth-smart products.
Tel: (03) 9690 9339
www.passionfoods.com.au

QUEENSLAND
Mrs Flannery's

Queensland's largest stockist of quality imported foods, as well as premium organically grown fruit and vegetables, whole foods, nuts, grains and cereals, flours and pastas, as well as herbs and spices. Shops throughout Queensland.
www.mrsflannerys.com.au

SOUTH AUSTRALIA
Real Organics

South Australia's largest organic super-market, stocking fresh fruit and vegeta-bles, wheat free/gluten free products, macrobiotic, vegan products and more. Real organics delivers Australia-wide.
Tel: (08) 8363 1911
www.realorganics.com.au

CHEMICAL-FREE SUNSCREENS
Avene Eau Thermale SPF30+ Sunscreen Cream 50ml

Avene is sold in most chemists throughout Australia.

Skin Ceuticals — Physical UV defense SPF 30 (90ml)

To find stockists or buy online go to www.superiorskincare.com.au

Clinique's SPF-25 Special Defense Sunblock

NEWSLETTERS, MAGAZINES AND PERIODICALS

Nature and Health — Bimonthly Australian magazine

A wonderful magazine for people inter-ested in maintaining a naturally healthy lifestyle. Beautifully illustrated features are presented in a highly attractive, informative and entertaining format. Topics include beauty, nutrition, healthy living, exercise, cooking and relationships. Available at newsagencies or by subscription.

Wellbeing — Quarterly Australian magazine

Wellbeing is a unique and respected natural health and lifestyle publication. With in-depth articles written by experts, each issue offers practical information and inspiration for the mind, body and soul.
www.wellbeing.com.au
Available at newsagencies or by sub-scription.

The Sinatra Health Report (online) by Dr Stephen Sinatra

A monthly newsletter focused on tips for increasing longevity and quality of life. www.drsinatra.com

The Health Sciences Institute Members Alert (online)

A cutting-edge newsletter delivered into your inbox daily and put out by a several top medical experts.
www.hsibaltimore.com

Dr Susan M. Lark's The Lark Letter: A Woman's Guide to Optimal Health and Balance (online)

This newsletter provides wonderful information on hormone-related weight issues, and all other health issues rele-vant to women.
www.drlark.com

Dr Joseph Mercola

Dr Mercola is the author of the *Total Health Program* and *The No Grain Diet*. He publishes an informative, free, twice-weekly health e-newsletter, which is loaded with health and wellness information. The site also has an excellent selection of products for online purchase. www.mercola.com

Life Extension magazine

Published by the Life Extension Foundation, this is arguably the most cutting-edge and informative online health resource. You need to sign up to become a member to receive their magazine. This will also allow you to receive discounts on their supplements. You don't have to be a member to log on for medical abstracts and medical protocols. www.lef.org

HEALTH SPAS / HEALTH RESORTS

The Springs

Hepburn Springs, Victoria
The Springs Retreat Boutique hotel and Mineral Spa located in Hepburn Springs offer an extensive range of relaxing and health-giving treatments (including hydrotherapy spas, chakra balancing, lymphatic drainage massage, massage, facials, shiatsu, deep tissue and reiki) in beautiful surroundings. Accommodation is a choice of 25 stylish rooms or spa suits. Yoga classes are also available.
Tel: (03) 5348 2202
www.thesprings.com.au

The Golden Door

Gold Coast, Queensland, and the Hunter Valley
www.goldendoor.com.au

Camp Eden

Gold Coast, Queensland
Both the Golden Door health retreat and Camp Eden offer excellent programs for health, wellbeing, relaxation and pampering. They both have an extensive range of treatments and therapies including acupuncture, naturopathy, nutrition, remedial and aromatherapy massage, body scrubs, oil wraps, hand and foot spas, personal counselling sessions, facials, and personal training. They also offer such activities as tennis, swimming, and golf. Guests also can learn stress management techniques such as meditation, Tai Chi, and yoga. They both offer specific programs such as rejuvenating yoga weeks and seven day detox programs regularly throughout the year. Please check their websites for further information. www.campeden.com.au

Kangaroo Island Health Retreat

Kangaroo Island Health Retreat is located on Kangaroo Island in South Australia and offers a variety of programs, including detoxification, pampering, weekend retreats and cooking and cleansing programs.
Tel: (08) 8553 5374
www.kihealthretreat.com

Further Reading

Aston Donna, *Staying Alive: Age-proof Your Body From the Inside Out*, Viking, Victoria, 2002.

Atkins Robert C., MD, *Dr Atkins' Age-Defying Diet*, St. Martin's Press, New York, 2001.

——, *Dr Atkins' New Diet Revolution*, New York: HarperCollins, 2002.

——, *Dr Atkins' Vita-Nutrient Solution: Nature's Answers to Drugs*, Fireside, New York, 1998.

Bland Jeffrey, PhD, *The 20-Day Rejuvenation Diet Program*, Keats Publishing, Connecticut, 1998.

Brand-Miller Jennie, Foster-Powell Kaye. *The New Glucose Revolution: The Glycaemic Index Solution for Optimum Health*, Hodder Headline, Sydney, 2000.

Challem Jack, *The Inflammation Syndrome*, John Wiley and Sons, New Jersey, 2003.

Chopra Deepak, MD, David Simon, *Grow Younger, Live Longer: Ten Steps to Reverse Ageing*, Three Rivers Press, New York, 2001.

Cochrane Amanda, *Perfect Skin: The Natural Approach*, Piatkus, London, 2000.

Cordain Loren, PhD, *The Paleo Diet: Lose Weight and Get Healthy by Eating the Food You Were Designed to Eat*, John Wiley and Sons, New York, 2002.

D'Adamo Peter J., *Eat Right for Your Type*, Putnam, New York, 1996.

——, *Live Right for Your Type: Four Blood Types*, Four Programs, Putnam, New York, 2001.

Elstein Michael MD, *Eternal Health*, Nacson and Sons, Sydney, 2000.

Enig Mary G., PhD, *Know Your Fats: The Complete Primer for Understanding the Nutrition of Fats, Oils and Cholesterol*, Bethesda Press, Maryland, 2003.

Erasmus Udo, *Fats That Heal, Fats That Kill: The Complete Guide to Fats, Oils, Cholesterol and Human Health*, Alice Books, Burnaby, B.C., Canada, 1993.

Erikson Kim, *Drop Dead Gorgeous*, Contemporary Books, Chicago, 2002.

Garcia Oz, *Look and Feel Fabulous Forever*, Regan Books, New York, 2002.

Giampapa Vincent, MD, Pero Ronald, PhD, and Zimmerman Marcia, *The Anti-aging Solution: Five Simple Steps to Looking and Feeling Young*, John Wiley and Sons, New Jersey, 2004.

Gittleman Anne Louise, *Get the Sugar Out: 501 Simple Ways to Cut the Sugar Out of Any Diet*, Three Rivers Press, New York, 1996.

——, *The Complete Fat Flush Program*. McGrawHill / Contemporary Books, New York, 2002.

——, *The Living Beauty Detox Program*, HarperSanFrancisco, New York, 2000.

Iyengar B. K. S., *Light on Yoga: The Bible of Modern Yoga*, Schocken Books, New York, 1995 (revised edition).

James Kat, *The Truth About Beauty: Transform Your Looks and Your Life From the Inside Out*. Beyond Words Publishing, Oregon, 2003.

Kenton Leslie, Age Power: *The Revolutionary Path to Natural High-tech Rejuvenation*, Random House, Sydney, 2002.

——, *Ten Steps to a Younger You*, Vermillion, London, 2000.

——, *The X Factor Diet: For Lasting Weight Loss and Vital Health*, Vermillion, London, 2002.

Kirsch David, *The Ultimate New York Body Plan: Just Two Weeks to a Total Transformation*, McGraw Hill, New York, 2004.

Kyriazis Marios, MD, *Stay Young, Longer Naturally: the Natural Anti-aging Plan*, Vega, London, 2001.

Murad Howard, *The Murad Method. Wrinkle-Proof, Repair and Renew Your Skin with the Proven 5-Week Program*, St Martins Press, New York, 2003.

Packer Lester, PhD, Coleman Carol, *The Antioxidant Miracle*, John Wiley & Sons, New York, 1999.

Perricone Nicolas, MD, *The Perricone Prescription*. HarperCollins, New York, 2002.

——, *The Perricone Promise: Look Younger, Live Longer in Three Easy Steps*, Warner Books, New York, 2004.

——, *The Wrinkle Cure: Unlock the Power of Cosmeceuticals for Supple, Youthful Skin*, Warner Books, New York, 2000.

Pitchford Paul, *Healing with Whole Foods: Oriental Traditions and Modern Nutrition*, North Atlantic Books, California, 1993.

Pratt Steven, MD, Mathews Kathy, *Superfoods: Fourteen Foods That Will Change Your Life*, Random House, Sydney, 2004.

Raichur Pratima, Cohn Marion Raichur, *Absolute Beauty: Radiant Skin and Inner Harmony through the Ancient Secrets of Ayurveda*, HarperCollins, New York, 1997.

Roizen Michael, MD, La Puma John, *The Real Age Diet: Make Yourself Younger with What You Eat*, HarperCollins, New York, 1999.

Roizen, Michael, MD, Oz, Mehmet, MD, *YOU: The Owner's Manual: An Insider's guide to the Body that Will Make You Healthier and Younger*, HarperResource, New York, 2005.

Rubin Jordan, PhD. *The Maker's Diet: The 40-day Health Experience That Will Change Your Life Forever*, Siloam, Florida, 2004.

Sears Barry, PhD, *A Week in the Zone*, Regan Books, New York, 2000.

——, *Enter the Zone*, Regan Books, New York, 1995.

———, *The Anti-aging Zone*, HarperCollins, New York, 1999.

Smith Timothy J., MD, Renewal: *The Anti-aging Revolution*, Rodale Press, Pennsylvania, 1998.

Somer Elizabeth, *The Origin Diet: How Eating Like Our Stone Age Ancestors Will Maximize Your Health*, Owl Books, New York, 2001.

Somers Suzanne, *The Sexy Years: Discover the Hormone Connection, the Secret to Fabulous Sex, Great Health, and Vitality, for Women and Men*, Crown, New York, 2004.

Sparrowe Linda, *Yoga: A Yoga Journal Book*, Hugh Lauter Levin Associates, Berkley, 2004.

Walford Roy, MD, *Beyond the 120 Year Diet: How to Double Your Vital Years*. Four Walls, Eight Windows, New York, 2000.

Weil Andrew, MD, *Eating Well for Optimum Health*. HarperCollins, New York, 2001.

Willcox Bradley, MD, Willcox Craig, PhD, and Suzuki Makoto, *The Okinawa Way: How to Improve Your Health and Longevity Dramatically*, Penguin, London, 2001.

Wolcott William, Fahey Trish, *The Metabolic Typing Diet*, Broadway Books, New York, 2000.

Index